The Bleeding Spine

The Bleeding Spine
. . .

Jim A. Larsen D.C.

© 2018 Jim A. Larsen D.C.
All rights reserved.

ISBN-13: 9781540793157
ISBN-10: 154079315X

Acknowledgements

● ● ●

Thanks to CreateSpace and Amazon for their expertise, editing and guidance to revise and publish my second literary effort.

I thank my loving and courageous late wife Romona who fought gracefully for a longer life and taught so many to be thankful for each day one receives.

I am grateful for my fiancée Isabel who inspires me daily and helps me balance my life.

I thank my families, my friends, and the patients who encouraged me to continue in my search of new ideas.

I am indebted to those whose lives have passed due to spinal trauma and a subsequent illness, let them not be forgotten. And for the survivors, may you continue to have passion for life and make it contagious for others.

This book is dedicated to Isabel's son Phillip, whose life ended way too soon at the age of fourteen. He is one of many who may have seeded cancer from an early childhood injury. We miss his smile and loving spirit.

Contents

Acknowledgements ... v
Author's Note ... ix
Preface ... xi
Introduction: Cancer and Autoimmune Disease: My Early Obsession ... xv

Chapter 1	Portrait of a Chiropractor's Injuries	1
Chapter 2	Genesis of My Theory	6
Chapter 3	Vertebral Compression Fracture	13
Chapter 4	Stem Cell: Creator, Culprit, and Cure	18
Chapter 5	Scoliosis and Kyphosis	23
Chapter 6	Intestinal Risks	28
Chapter 7	Heart and Lung Disease	39
Chapter 8	Melanoma and Brain Tumors	45
Chapter 9	Multiple Sclerosis and Aortic Aneurysm	49
Chapter 10	Medications, Osteoporosis, and Spontaneous Vertebral Compression Fractures	53
Chapter 11	Breast Cancer	57
Chapter 12	Multiple Myeloma and Leukemia	59
Chapter 13	Cranium and Brain Trauma	62
Chapter 14	Colostrum: First Immune Codes	65
Chapter 15	Prevention and Immunotherapy	69

Author's Note

• • •

THE INFORMATION CONTAINED IN THIS book is based upon the author's personal experiences and observation, as well as researching medical, radiological, and contemporary experimental research by professionals throughout the world. All publications and Internet sources of information used in this book have been obtained from public domain.

The material in this book is for informational purposes only. It is not intended to be or serve as a substitute for consultation with your personal physician and/or health care provider. The publisher, author, and/or experts cited in this publication are not responsible for and consequences, direct or indirect, resulting from any reader's actions.

The purpose of this publication is to educate the reader as to a generalized theory of possible outcomes from vertebral compression fractures. To protect their privacy, names have been changed for the individual patients mentioned in this book, and in some instances, biographical details about them has been altered. The author has no financial interest in any companies that produce, market, sell, or distribute products mentioned in the book.

Preface

Time to head back to the original title

My first book "Stem Cells and Spinal Trauma" introduced my 1985 theory that stem cells are seeds of cancer and autoimmune disease when set free from the interior of red bone marrow. For the first twenty years, my patients and friends were told of the original title for this book as "The Bleeding Spine". I promised my deceased wife Romona I would someday write the book, and that this would be the title. However, during the professional help of writing the first book, the editor suggested I include "stem cells" in the title. This has led to my first book being lost due to the voluminous promotion of stem cell research and treatment promises.

We now live in an age where more than half the population uses the internet daily and the use of cell phones, smart or not, takes the time and attention of millions of people across the globe. Want to know something? Look it up! I found out the use of the Internet for searching medical or scientific information has a plethora of opinions by professionals and non-professionals. The information age appears to be controlled by medical institutions and for their own gain. So, typing into your screen the words "stem cells" leads you to seven million articles. Now try to get past the first six million articles. The too numerous articles that promise the supposed benefits of stem cell treatments. You would be lucky to find my book title. Search deep enough and you will find articles that truthfully relay the proven dangers of stem cell treatment and use.

A chiropractor theorizing and writing a book about a crazy idea that stem cells may be a cause of cancer seems far-fetched. And to use the term stem cells within the title sounds overly scientific. I had reservations about this new title, after all, I had told over a thousand people for twenty years that the title would be The Bleeding Spine. Maybe this mistake was meant to be as I promote the new book by adding my x-rays, new information and more living examples.

Along my most recent search on stem cells brought forth the studies from 1855 by a German pathologist named Rudolf Virchow. He had proposed that cancers arise from the activation of dormant, embryonic-like cells present in mature tissue. My theory deals with the bleeding of immature stem cells from the red bone marrow into the nerves and tissues. I correlated traumatic spinal fractures with illnesses. My observations were more on the outside looking in. I didn't need a microscope to see an illness. Just a good weight bearing x-ray. My patients understood that I was always searching for the **cause** of cancer. I was never interested in the cure for cancer. The far more common interest regards the **cure** for cancer. Most scientists would agree, that understanding of the cause of cancer will help lead to the cure of cancer.

This time The Bleeding Spine has the correct title, has become a renewed reality, and hopefully it's revision has a better chance to reach the science community and openly gain some public interest. I can't believe how the substantial amount of research released that exposes the serious side effects of stem cell use has been cloaked over so extensively that even the FDA cannot keep pace with the clinics and treatment centers portraying falsely the promise of stem cell benefits. The companies that have the money can push their false promises to the top of the list on internet search. I find the overall public does not have a clue to the fact that original and continued research reveals that the use and application of stem cells in treatment of disease have a long way to go to get past the serious side effects that stem cell use produces.

The mainstream information I provide in The Bleeding Spine still expounds on the ill effects that develop when trauma produces a bleeding out of the undeveloped cells of the hematopoietic or red bone marrow system. The bleeding releases stem like cellular materials so small that they should not be called a cell. Trauma to the red bone marrow includes not only the damage to mature cells, but a release of the stored and dormant inaugural genetic codes that gave the very birth to those cells. These materials or protein codes are inaugural progenitors that should never leave their contained environment until histologically developed into a cell. Spinal trauma produces a code leakage, a sort of epigenetic flow which later becomes an immune engulfed genetic expression. The message behind The Bleeding Spine is to remind the community that our bodies may contain a mechanism of self-destruction that is just a natural system of physiology. Did our Creator goof up? Is our immune system so vulnerable that it absorbs its creator codes and then is altered to war against the very body that supports it? Just doesn't seem right that the very system that protects our health, stabs us in the back (no pun intended). Yet it truly happens to millions of folks in in thousands of ways. There will be a never-ending list of new and rare diseases and cancer as there is the never-ending potential of combinations of bleeding of genetic codes.

I put out a question on Yahoo in 2012 a year before I published Stem Cells and Spinal Trauma. I asked the public: "Have you ever had a vertebral compression fracture that had led to autoimmune disease or cancer?" I received very little response. However, one reply found the theory "Interesting "and replied "Compression fracture of the spine is often caused by the cancer or immune disease not the other way around." The reply remarked "Often injury is the first indicator that the disease was there (I. E. The disease preexisted the injury – not the other way around). The reply continues "Stem cells don't cause illness." "Your theory is flawed." Guess this person never read the original findings on stem cell research.

The Bleeding Spine tells the story of my observations of seven hundred to eight hundred people who develop cancer or autoimmune disease **after** vertebral fracture. Yes, most of the cases develop problems months to many years later following the injury – but a sizable portion of the cases went into a serious disease state immediately after the trauma. None of the seven hundred plus cases I observed had a pre-diagnosis of any disease. There is a specific reason to why this happened. I presented an article on my theory to patients, friends, and family in 1985. It explained my request and search for subjects that have had a vertebral compression fracture that **preceded any diagnosis of illness,** and yet had ended up in cancer or autoimmune disease post-injury. My theory and the article even ended up across our country. A grand search was started to find out if trauma to the axial skeleton with the bleeding of stem cells from the red bone marrow, would produce cancer or autoimmune disease.

I was amazed how my crazy idea supported itself through simple observation on a spinal x-ray. No microscope needed here. Just follow up on the falling, crunching population that crack a skull, break a posterior vertebral arch or compress vertebral bodies together. Every case of traumatic fracture I have examined has eventual developed disease. The trauma outcomes repetitively revealed a direct relationship to the nearby nerves that absorbed up the bleeding inaugural codes and ended up changing the connective tissue of the organ they innervated. What was announced in September 2003 simply amazed and overwhelmed me! After hundreds of injury cases in my collection, in 2003 scientists announced that (cancer) stem cells are the cause and seeding of up to 70% of cancer types in the human body.

I had never sought the academic review of my work and findings by anyone. Local medical doctors were amazed at my findings. I never wrote a peer-reviewed article for a couple of reasons. One, I had my own reservations about my observations even though hundreds of my patients who fell victim to cancer stem cells sure believed in my theory. Secondly, I needed time to love and care for a wife who had lost her kidneys due to auto-immune disease. True love sets true priorities. When you read The Bleeding Spine, keep in mind a young boy taking an interest primarily in the **cause** of cancer, who later conjured up a crazy theory that stem cells escape marrow, penetrate and flow down nerves and up spinal fluids and enter lung and abdomen cavities. The stem cells then embed into the connective tissues and organs as a seed, a virus, an undeveloped code, soon engulfed by its own immune cell offspring. Mutations occur and quickly or insidiously altering the codes of growing cells nearby, producing an army of antibodies against its own, and infusing the code of repetitive cell growth, to become cancer.

INTRODUCTION

Cancer and Autoimmune Disease: My Early Obsession

● ● ●

HAVE YOU EVER BEEN OBSESSED with something? So much that it sticks in your mind and haunts you endlessly? How about the cause of cancer? Wouldn't it be fabulous to come up with a solution to something that causes so much suffering and loss of life? Scientists around the globe contemplate possible answers, studying diseased cells under microscopes in a race to save a patient, a loved one or even their own lives.

I have been obsessed with cancer since I was a ten-year-old boy. It first started when I visited my sweet Grandma weeks before her frail, cancer-ridden body failed. Growing up, books and encyclopedias surrounded me in my bedroom converted from a den. I started to search for answers to cancer in any book I could get my hands on. My search centered on the cause of cancer. I didn't have much interest in the treatment of cancer. I still believe understanding to cause of cancer will lead to improved treatment and better prevention.

Cancer plagued our family and close friends. My mother lost her mom and best friend to cancer. My best friend across the street lost his father and then his sister to cancer when we were twelve years old. My Uncle loss his life due to stomach cancer. I needed answers. The information I read talked about a malfunctioning immune system, blood and lymph fluids carrying cancer cells. Metastasis was everywhere. Cells mutated and traveled. Tumors appeared as diseased cells grew out of control.

Cancer theories shifted as years went by. Fluid theories dropped off, and studies focused on cells. Carcinogens, toxins, x-rays, ultraviolet light and industrial wastes disrupted cells. I never believed that only these factors caused cell mutation. I kept searching for new ideas.

My young life of studying cancer, its cause and treatment, kept rolling after I fell in love with a young woman whose kidneys were failing. My keen interest in cancer expanded to include autoimmune disease, where the body's immune cells attack its own cells and tissues. In these early studies I came to realize that autoimmune disease and cancer is initiated at the connective tissues or base framework layer of an organ. This is the site where our immune starts the disease, the base continual growing type tissues. In heart disease, kidney disease, aortic aneurysm and dilatation of bowel tissue, the connective tissue is where the tissue loss or tissue gain is occurring. Even myelin coverings of spinal cord and nerves are attacked and devoured by our own immune system. Immune cells are drawn to the framework tissue of the body — the collagen-based connective tissue. Rarely do immune cells attack specialized cells such as muscle, heart, nerve, and liver cells.

In 1985, a patient I was examining told me he had recently had a portion of his colon removed due to cancer. He was 50 years old and worked hard as a rancher. I took x-rays to investigate his lower back pain. What I saw on his spinal x-rays matched up with the nerves that innervate the colon. The lumbar spine had a lateral compression trauma at the first two lumbar vertebrae. Recently I had learned at research seminars that nerves exhibit protein flow down their axon pathways. I thought, what small entity could travel down the nerves to invoke cancer or autoimmune disease? What I about stem cells or DNA material. Stem cells are very small genetic coded proteins. These tiny cells are the smallest protein molecules in the body. Could they penetrate and pass into autonomic nerves and travel downstream to organ tissues?

The scientific models for nerve interference were changing after I graduated in 1979. The bigger picture was driven inward with research findings coming from a molecular level. Studies were proving that leg pain was due more to absorption of small inflammatory proteins than to compressed nerves, and that proteins can flow down the axon or center of a nerve into organs of the body. Today researchers are studying the use of nerves as a vector for drug therapy to the tissues. Stem cells are the smallest strands of genetic protein to initiate the growth of a cell. Could something as small as a stem cell are stem cell debris be involved in inflaming organs and tissues?

Then it came to me. Stem cells are exceedingly small protein strands that contain DNA codes. They also contain the self-renewal codes to replicate themselves and codes that the use to differentiate into mature tissues. I thought, stem cells if raw and undeveloped, may resemble viruses and can absorb into, pass through, and migrate along nerves. Protected within nerve pathways, stem cells particles can avoid an immune system attack and can easily flow into the framework tissues of organs.

In 1985 I wrote a patient handout about my idea of stem cells invoking autoimmune disease and cancer. I began to look for a population of people who had developed illness **after** trauma to the spine that involved vertebral compression fracture. I was looking for the injuries that **preceded** any diagnosis of illness. My wife and I have large agricultural families that have lived in the same town for decades. It was easy to find ranchers, farmers and horseback riders who had suffered fall-type injuries that compressed their spines.

My family and patients listened and believed in what I had to say. Cases of vertebral compression fracture with associated illness after the injury started to come in. The vertebral fractures had led to patterns of illness corresponding to the location of nearby organs or those that could be reached by stem cells traveling down nearby nerve pathways. The same fracture levels kept resulting in the same types of illnesses. My idea of spinal damage involvement in the development of cancer and autoimmune disease was evolving as my wife's health declined. My experience surrounding her autoimmune disease of her kidneys taught me multitudes about the illness. My love and energy also went into caring for her until her death in 2011.

These stories and patients are real. Stem cells cause illness. Type any disease into your computer search engine, follow it with the words, "stem cells," and you'll see what I mean. You may have to scroll deep past numerous treatment articles to find causation articles. This book describes selected stories out of nearly 700 patients from my chiropractic practice to illustrate how vertebral compression fractures lead to illness. The following introductory story is a common and good example of what I have observed for the past thirty-five years. Keep in mind that most of the patients in this book are relatives and close friends of mine. I just may have been in the right place at the right to learn an unnoticed way that people become ill.

Erika's Fall from Sugar

Erika worked in town but loved to spend time at her two-acre property caring for her garden and her horse, Sugar. She would spend afternoons after work and weekends riding Sugar through the rolling hills and oaks above her property. One day, in a gentle gallop, a rattlesnake startled Sugar. The horse reared up in fear, throwing Erika from the saddle. Sugar came back to her unhurt, but it was not the same for her rider and caretaker. Erika's fall to the rocky ground lead to several serious illnesses and would ruin her life.

About a week after the riding accident, Erika called for a chiropractic appointment at my office. She told me about the fall off Sugar. Back pain restricted her freedom of movement. I gently realigned her vertebrae and provided traction and myofascial massage to her strained spinal muscles. She improved and stabilized within two weeks of initial treatment, and I released her to schedule wellness appointments.

Initially I treated Erika for her pain and restriction in her lower back and neck. She returned for another appointment about three months later. Erika had been diagnosed with breast cancer by her doctor. The news brought us both to tears. Erika had been a patient of mine for almost fifteen years. She knew of my theory linking compression fractures with autoimmune disease and cancer. I suggested an x-ray of her back to look for compression fractures, but she resisted, worried about the risk of radiation. I asked Erika to continue treatment at my office, so I could follow the outcome of this injury and her health.

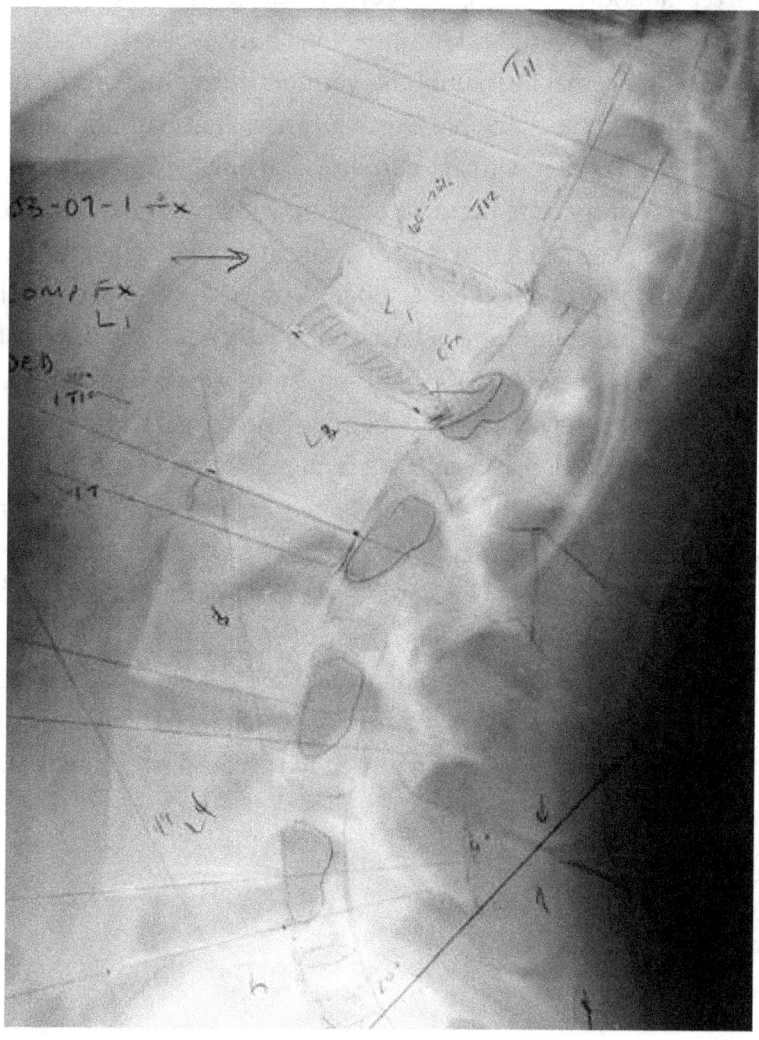

A few weeks later, Erika allowed the doctor to remove the cancerous breast. After the mastectomy, she continued to go to a nearby medical center for weekly chemotherapy. I continued examining and treating her each week. Then one-week Erika came in with more sad news. Her doctor had ordered a CT and x-rays on her body. The images revealed a crushing fracture to the first lumbar vertebrae of her spine. We were now both in tears again. Scans that were taken also revealed growths or tumors that developed in her liver, kidneys, and intestines. Cancer had invaded the entire region near the initial spinal fracture from the horse accident: the 11th and 12th thoracic vertebrae and the first lumbar vertebra. These vertebrae are associated with nerves supplying organs and tissues of both the thoracic and abdominal cavities of our body. Erika's health began to fade rapidly in the ensuing months as disease took over and destroyed her tissues.

Erika also complained of headaches over the course of her weekly treatment. I corrected the region around her upper cervical vertebrae with gentle settings as she lay on her side. Treatment was helpful in relieving her neck pain, headaches, and lower back pain, giving Erika some relief over the months. During a routine visit she complained of a headache. Upon examination I found no subluxation of her upper cervical vertebrae. She was holding her alignment from the week before. I explained that her recent headaches were not caused from vertebral misalignment. Within a week of this appointment, her doctor ordered an MRI of her brain. The brain scan revealed that Erika had several brain tumors! The original bleeding stem cells from her accident had penetrated the spinal cord covering, entered the cerebrospinal fluids and ascended to her brain. The blood supply on the outside of the brain is an easy target for the seeding of stem cells.

Erika lived about a year and a half after falling off Sugar. Her case is far from unusual. Her injuries and subsequent illness fit a pattern of more than 700 patients and family I have examined over the course of thirty-eight years as a chiropractor. My practice is in horse and dairy country north of San Francisco. Many of my patients suffer injuries from car accidents, horseback riding falls, or falls and lifting injuries due to taking care of cows, sheep, and poultry. The injuries that have especially caught my interest involve a lateral compression injury to the vertebral body. These injuries correlate with an onset of initial inflammation, and autoimmune type disease. In some cases, the vertebral compression injury evolved quickly into cancer of an organ. These people were healthy and living normal lives, until the vertebral compression fracture occurred. The fracture did not occur because of metastatic cancer or pre-existing cancer that had not yet been diagnosed. In these stories, spinal injuries led directly and often swiftly to autoimmune disease and cancer.

Erika's story tops them all. She knew my theory for over fifteen years from the article I had handed out to patients since 1985. I had already associated over three hundred cases of vertebral fracture injury with possible stem cell leakage when her accident occurred. I had seen similar fractures at levels of the spine with repeated evidence of autoimmune disease and/or cancer. I was worried about Erika at the onset of her injury. She had poor healing ability from factors that I consistently associated with a cancer outcome, instead of autoimmune disease. She did not receive colostrum as an infant, a major association to evolving cancer. Ericka was a vegan for thirty years. She was also a smoker. In coming chapters I will tell stories of patients and acquaintances of mine who became ill after fractures of the vertebral body, sacrum, and ribs. Along with compression fracture, moderate intervertebral disc herniation and chance fracture also can bleed stem cells.

In the next chapter I will explain in more detail how the idea of red bone marrow leakage causing illness came to me in 1985. Erika not only knew of my stem cell leakage theory, she knew of some of the stories of others before her who have had spinal injury and developed into illness. Her unfortunate injury and the eventual outcome provide evidence of my theory of stem cells bleeding from a fracture and developing into a serious illness. Most of the patient cases presented in this book are friends and family members who I have known for years.

CHAPTER 1

Portrait of a Chiropractor's Injuries

• • •

ONE DAY WHEN I WAS five years old, I was riding in the backseat of my dad's 1956 Chevy station wagon. An athletic boy, I usually preferred to be on my feet – running, playing, or climbing rather than sitting in a car. In those days cars did not have seatbelts. Squeezed into the backseat next to my four sisters, I was frustrated with an uncomfortable car ride. My shoulder was pressed up against the side of the door as my father drove down the road. I accidentally elbowed the side door handle, and the door flew open. I lost my balance and tumbled onto the roadway. My dad had no time to brake as the right rear tire of the Chevy hit my head. The impact caused severe pain around my temple and forehead, later evolving into chronic neck pain and migraine headaches. The left side of my head and eye region turned black and blue for weeks, until gradually the injuries began to heal, at least on the surface.

As a young student I experienced migraine headaches so severe that they nearly incapacitated me with blinding pain. More than once I passed out, the pain was so horrendous. The back of my head on the left side was always in pain, and when one of the migraine headaches settled in, I could barely open my eyes. During my elementary school years, the left side of my face was tight and distorted. My smile and my head tipped upward on the left. Pain frequently visited the back of my head and neck. Several times I ended up vomiting from the pain.

Also, during these years, I experienced profound nausea. Carsickness was inevitable. Even a short ride on a merry-go-round would upset my stomach or make me severely dizzy. There were times during my youth when I was extremely sensitive to light. White flashes would appear in my sight during a migraine headache. My jaw would lock up and become tight if I chewed gum. Migraine headaches plagued me monthly for nearly forty-five years. With no medical intervention, I survived this ordeal, withstood the pain, and came to understand it from the point of view of a patient. Despite regular bouts of agony, I was profoundly fortunate. My brain made it through the accident without apparent damage, though it may have caused a chronic condition of hyperactivity. I felt the need to move my body constantly. Scar tissue formed which tightened my vertebrae and locked them out of alignment for years.

Young bodies have enormous benefits when it comes to recovery from injury. Abundant growth hormones swirl through the body's tissues. The body forms collagen, bone, and cells at rapid rates. The growth factors of a child's body are prepared for the inevitable mishaps of youth. During puberty and the years of growth hormone, a young person's body heals quite readily. An injury in youth heals much better than an injury as an adult, or as an infant. School studies came easily for me, and I was grateful to find my memory and intellectual gifts intact. By the time I finished middle school, I graduated as valedictorian of my class, and in high school I graduated with honors. With the hindsight of over thirty years of chiropractic work, I have no doubt that the fall out of the car likely twisted my neck and permanently damaged the suboccipital and other neck muscles attached to the upper two of my seven cervical vertebrae.

Bike crash

Other accidents aggravated the structure of my young growing spine. One day I rode my Schwinn Western Flyer bike to school after a piano lesson. As I peddled down the corridor between classrooms, I noticed other boys riding on their stingray bikes from the cement corridor out onto the lawn and then launching themselves into the air on a plywood ramp. That looked exciting and fun. So, I borrowed one of their bikes, pumped hard on the pedals, picked up speed and hit the ramp. I had not noticed that the other boys would pop up their front wheels just as they hit the ramp to propel themselves upward.

The bike's front wheel hit the ramp and got stuck. The bike stopped, and I flew over the handlebars with my arms outstretched as if I were training to be an eagle. The flight ended badly. I crashed headfirst into the grass onto my chin, hyper-extending my neck as I slid ten or fifteen feet along the grass. No doubt that trauma further damaged all the vertebrae of my neck.

Fall from tree

As an avid tree climber, filled with more ambition than caution, one day I ascended to the upper branches of a live oak tree. Up high where the branches were slender, I kept climbing, fearless in my ascent toward the clouds. I loved the feeling of being high off the ground. Without warning, the branch that held my left foot snapped and I plummeted to the ground. I fell feet first, smashing my left leg into the hard ground, luckily not breaking any bones. Falling to one side, my lower spine folded or twisted on impact, causing compression damage to the lumbar region of my spine. God had smiled on me once more and pulled me through with my brain intact. Had I tumbled headfirst to the ground, I could easily have broken my neck or fractured my skull. My career as a chiropractor would never have happened.

The tree accident most likely caused an initial intervertebral disc injury in my lower back at my fifth lumbar vertebra. My young body received a new pattern of pain in my lower back and left leg. After a few months of healing, my leg was ready for more action. My spirit emerged unscathed. Soon I was eager to go. With unusually speedy feet, I started playing soccer in elementary school, in the defensive fullback position. I could often outrun competing offensive players to kick the ball away from them and prevent them from scoring goals.

When I reached middle school, a coach encouraged me to try out for track. For six years I competed as a sprinter. Running fast was more exciting to me than running long distances. Here again my eagerness to compete led me to exceed my body's limits. Each year of track I struggled with the same afflictions: spasms in my lower back, left hip pain and constant contraction of my left hamstring muscles. My left lower back suffered from the forces of running. My left sciatic nerve was irritated due to the instability of my lower back discs.

In nearly every race, I was fast enough to lead most runners in the pack for the first stretch. However, in the final sprint of the race, my lower back and left leg would tighten up so severely that other competitors would pass me before the finish line. It was as though giant tethers grabbed me from behind and tugged my body into a rigid, painful plank. Sometimes I could not even finish the race. Though I had the speed to excel as one of the faster athletes, pain inhibited my potential. I knew I could do better. It didn't help that during longer races on the track runners always lean to the left into counterclockwise turns. Hamstring problems tend to plague track runners and baseball players on the left side due to sprinting counterclockwise and leaning the spine to the left.

SEVERE AUTOMOBILE ACCIDENT

In 1972, just a few months before I was to graduate high school, my encounters with physical injury and pain made a sharp turn for the worse. One Friday in late December, my friend and classmate Michael suggested that we drive his 1968 Mercury Capri to the UC Berkeley library to research term papers for an English class we had together. That Friday night I had a vivid dream that Michael and I were in a bad car accident together. When I woke up Saturday, I told my mother about the dream and she cautioned me to be careful on the trip. Michael and I drove to Berkeley without incident, but the library was closed for winter break. We wandered around the campus for a while then decided to drive across the Bay Bridge to San Francisco before heading back home.

As we headed down Highway 880, traffic was crowded but moving at a steady sixty-five miles an hour. I noticed I had only fastened my lap belt and forgot to attach my shoulder belt. In cars of that vintage, shoulder and seat belts were separate. So, I turned and pulled the shoulder belt out and clicked its buckle into the latch. Within seconds, a car further up the line in front of us swerved into our lane and the driver two cars in front of us slammed on his brakes. A Ford LTD in front of us also braked hard but collided. Michael reacted a split second too late and our car's small narrow tires lost their grip on the roadway. We slid and plowed into the back of the LTD.

In quick succession, two cars behind us slammed into our rear. We were sandwiched between four cars! Within a couple of seconds, we had sustained three impacts at speeds exceeding sixty miles an hour. Dazed we lay sprawled in the Capri at the center of this five-car destruction derby. The impact forced my car seat backward. The trunk collapsed from the rear impact and crumpled into the seat that cradled my head. Our car, hit once from the front and twice in the back, had transformed from a sporty auto into a twisted, jagged pile of torn metal and plastic, littered with broken glass.

Looking over at Michael, I notice he had been forced into the steering wheel by the impact, and probably cracked some ribs. Miraculously the car could still move so Michael drove it to the shoulder of the highway. In shock and utterly disoriented, we dragged ourselves from the wreckage and staggered around on the pavement. We were alone on the freeway shoulder as the other four vehicles were able to pull off at an exit.

A highway patrol officer arrived and asked if we were okay. We were in no position to assess our physical condition, but we both nodded yes. A tow truck hauled Michael's wrecked Capri to an Oakland junkyard while we rode with him in the cab. We noticed several other Capris of similar model year with major damage at the junkyard. One car had its windshield broken through with blood splattered across the hood. The tow truck driver told us the Capri's driver, a young woman, had been thrown through the windshield and killed in the accident. While fun to drive, small cars had undersized narrow tires whose grip on the pavement was inadequate during sudden braking. Still discombobulated, we counted ourselves blessed to be alive.

We boarded a city bus in Oakland intending to find our way back to Sonoma County. While riding in the bus, I had a powerful premonition that we were heading for another accident. Seconds later a small car pulled directly in front of the bus, causing the bus plow into the car. The impact sent bus passengers flying toward the front of the bus. When the bus driver asked us to fill out injury cards, we laughed and said we were almost killed in an accident an hour earlier. Jostled, and not knowing if we were further injured, we transferred to another bus, and finally we were able to make it home.

Though I was grateful to be alive, my body was not happy with the events of that day. The migraine headaches and neck pain I had suffered since tumbling out of my dad's car intensified. Some days I wished, honestly, that I had not survived. Herniated discs in my lower neck shot pain into my neck and upper back. At times the pain was moderate to severe. I remember being in daily pain through the remainder of my senior year at high school. Pain can really drag you down.

The injuries inflamed my nerves, and I lost feeling in my hands and arms. The mechanical work I had enjoyed doing on my Ford Model A became excruciating torture. My head and arms felt heavy and my strength dwindled because of pain. The auto accident led to further injury to my left lower back. The lower back pain produced spasms and searing pain in my left hip and leg. At times the pain radiated all the way to the foot. I could not sit, stand, or lie down without provoking pain and spasms. Even the skin on my left leg showed signs of irritation, with bouts of psoriasis. Trauma to my lower lumbar discs produced chronic inflammation in my low back, pelvis, and left leg.

Within six months of the accident I had spinal x-rays taken at the hospital and visited an orthopedic surgeon. Because he knew my parents, he did not examine me. He reviewed the x-ray images then looked me squarely in the eye. The orthopedist pronounced, "There isn't a damn thing wrong with your x-rays. You're only eighteen. Live with it!" So, I did, while wondering to myself: this was medical care? What an astonishingly crass bedside manner.

A few years after our crash, Michael had another car accident where he again cracked ribs when striking the steering wheel. While I was studying in Chiropractic College I learned that he had died of lung lymphoma cancer at age 24, possibly because of leaked stem cells from one or both accidents. I was honored to serve as a pallbearer for his funeral.

Migraines and back pain tormented me as a young adult. In junior college I continued pre-medical courses to become a physical therapist. When I played junior college soccer, I was a starter, even though my back and leg would go into painful spasms, and I would have to leave the game to stretch. My neck, back, and leg pain impeded my studies and temporarily ruined my ability to learn. My grades declined to a C average because I could not recall what I studied due to bouts of pain. I broke pencils in anger during exams because the pain ruined my memory and my concentration. Even sitting in a chair for an entire hour was beyond my ability. My capacity to remember facts had eroded.

A new window was about to open. One of my classmates in chemistry suggested that I seek help from a chiropractor. I went to a local chiropractor, who observed that my injuries included a classic whiplash, hyperextension injury, ligament tears and vertebral subluxation. The chiropractor said my pain and inflammation was related to abnormal immobility and misalignment of vertebrae and discs of my upper and lower spine. Subluxation is not as severe as a dislocation, but the inflammation produces pain and inflammatory proteins that interfere with nerve function. My chiropractor's treatments gradually helped control the pain, which allowed me to regain functionality that I otherwise would have lost. My college grades soon went back to A's, and my memory function excelled.

Inspired by my chiropractor's talents, wisdom and how natural chiropractic works, I changed my major and went on to study at Palmer College of Chiropractic in Davenport, Iowa. I earned my doctorate degree, graduated in 1979, and launched my own practice in my hometown. I took extra courses at Palmer and became certified in the Grostic method of precision adjustments of the upper cervical region. The technique focuses on misalignment of the first and second cervical vertebrae, also called the atlas and axis, located at the base of the skull. The technique aims to alleviate irritation of the spinal cord in this region, which can cause myriad illnesses including migraines, dizziness, whole spine contraction and cranial neuritis.

The Grostic Upper Cervical method uses a manual hands-on technique of providing a light thrust to the vertebrae without affecting the head or other sections of the spine. This high-velocity but low-amplitude adjustment may occur in a region of less than half an inch while the patient is in a side posture position. The healing effect can be profound after a few sessions as the vertebrae revert to their normal positions and motion. Three-dimensional x-rays help to guide treatments with precision using measured line drawings that provide vectors and angles to adjust the vertebrae.

At Palmer College of Chiropractic, I studied many approaches to spinal care that allow me to safely release the vertebrae into a healthy position. Over the first fifteen years I studied and practiced Dr. James Cox's technique of flexion distraction for disc protrusions. Dr. Cox redesigned an osteopathic table for traction of the spine in a manual flexion manner. The specialized equipment and hands-on manual traction works especially well on disc protrusions where the disc folds outward due to injury or degeneration. Spinal manipulation is applied first to the vertebrae to release them into position. The treatment continues with flexion traction and long axis traction to open space between spinal segments. The manual contact on the vertebrae helps invert the protruding disc and increases the disc height. Even a 10-millimeter protrusion can recede entirely and heal back into place. Surrounding nerves often resume functioning. With this form of treatment, patients experience a slight increase in their overall height.

Problems with the lumbar discs of my back persisted for nearly twenty years until new research was discovered on what nutritionally heals the intervertebral disc. Chiropractic treatments, spinal research, and nutrition to grow collagen all improved and vitalized my life. To live free of migraine headaches has been phenomenally uplifting for my personal outlook. My left leg has regained most of the strength that I did not have for years. Most of this rebound in my own body came from my diet. I will explain why it is so important to have daily essential sulfur amino acids in your diet in Chapter 15 — Prevention and Immunotherapy — what it takes to improve your immune system and promote fast and continuous healing. I believe all other medical and natural approaches to healing will work if doctors and practitioners realize the importance of the sulfur-carbon bond. It's great having no pain and feeling better as one gets older. All the population of people who have lived well past one hundred years have one thing in common-they had a lifetime diet of the essential sulfur amino acids.

CHAPTER 2

Genesis of My Theory

● ● ●

DISEASE QUEST: FOR THE LOVE OF GRANDMA

When illness strikes at home, it hits deep in the heart. The first time my brain was in a quandary over cancer was at age ten after my grandmother Nana had fallen ill and died of kidney cancer. I was shocked and dismayed when I visited her once before she passed away. Her pale, thin and frail body left an image that scarred my mind. Then my mom's best friend, my Uncle Dale and my dad's best died from cancer. Then my best friend's sister succumbed to cancer in her early twenties. Cancer surrounded our neighborhood. From that point forward, I wanted to learn all I could about cancer. Science and biology were favorite subjects. As a child I read avidly about cancer and diseases, and I was always surprised that medical research could never fully explain the cause. As a young adult, I would look up theories on cancer as I progressed through my pre-medical courses in high school and junior college.

MORE CLUES: MY WIFE'S KIDNEY DISEASE

On our initial date, my wife to-have told me that both of her kidneys were failing due to an autoimmune disease known as acute glomerulonephritis. The condition affects renal function as an immunologic mechanism causing inflammation and degeneration of kidney tissue. Her own immune system was attacking her kidneys. As my chiropractic practice continued to thrive, I learned about my wife's kidney illness. I sought to help her survive. Some researchers attribute the disease to a virus or bacteria invading the kidneys, though this was never conclusively determined. Treatment for glomerulonephritis is primarily supportive; there is no cure.

Autoimmune disease in the kidneys attacks the interstitial or framework tissue of the organ. My wife's kidneys were losing function as the immune system eroded their structural components made of collagen. As I studied about her predicament on a personal quest to help her, I discovered research that helped me form a theory that involved the bleeding of marrow stem cells and how they can lead to illness. My interest gained momentum as I went on to absorb volumes of information on other autoimmune diseases, along with heart disease and cancer. My wife's illness affected us profoundly and provoked me to keep searching for answers.

Leo's Colon Cancer

As a shipyard worker, Leo worked hard for more than 30 years at the Bay Area docks. He was stocky and strong, 50 years old when he sought care at my chiropractic office. In Leo's first interview, he complained of a long history of lower back pain, especially on his left side. He had had recent surgery for colon cancer. I took standing x-rays of his lower back. An old trauma caught my eye as soon as the film dried. Leo had a large lateral disc protrusion between vertebrae lumbar two and lumbar three. It looked as if the entire disc was pushed out to the left margins of the vertebrae. The left top side of the L2 vertebral body was compressed by the bottom left side of the L1 vertebral body. A lateral compression injury took place. The healing response to the blown-out disc formed a thick seal of calcium deposits outside the large left disc protrusion. His body healed with incredible mineralization. Why did his injury heal this way?

On the next visit, Leo and I went over his x-rays together. He had an old compression injury to the left side of his lower back. I told him that it was a past injury where he must have been folded over to the left and compressed the upper two lumbar vertebrae together. He told me of an injury where he had slipped and fallen off the upper deck of a ship and landed on his leg and back on a lower platform. His back had been hurting him ever since.

An idea came to me while I was treating Leo's spine. The large disc protrusion to the outside of the two vertebrae is at a location where sympathetic nerves have their beginning pathways. In fact, the autonomic nerve passes directly along the side and the upper half of the vertebral body. An injury of this magnitude would have inflamed this nerve immediately after the accident. I asked Leo if it was the descending portion of the colon that had been removed due to cancer. He said yes. Now my mind started ticking with renewed vigor; I wanted to correlate his injury with his cancer.

Lateral Compression Fracture

The drawing and x-ray images below reveal a lateral type compression fracture to the vertebral body. In acute trauma, stem cells and disrupted red marrow matrix will bleed out adjacent to the sympathetic nerve at the side of collapse. Can stem cells and microcells penetrate a damaged nerve and flow down the axon? The recent trials of applying medications directly to diseased organs via nerves by injection may just provide the answer.

Over thirty years ago, research discovered that nerves have small proteins that flow down the axon and into the tissues. I believe injecting nerve axons with stem cells will develop diseases such as Shingles, Crohn's, Ulcerative colitis, Endometriosis, and cancers such as Colon, Bladder, and Pancreas. Injury to the same spinal segment on different individuals has led to the same organ disease state with those individuals.

The patient whose x-ray is viewed had a traumatic fall early in his life that crushed the lumbar vertebrae. He started out with bowel problems and ended up in later life with colon cancer. I have seen this very scenario two hundred times in my practice. Colon cancer linked to injury is one of the most common observations I have made, due to the fact the first two lumbar vertebrae are the most common compression fractures due to falls. Their position is under the thoracic spine which is more inflexible and thrusts into the first lumbar vertebra during a fall to the tailbone.

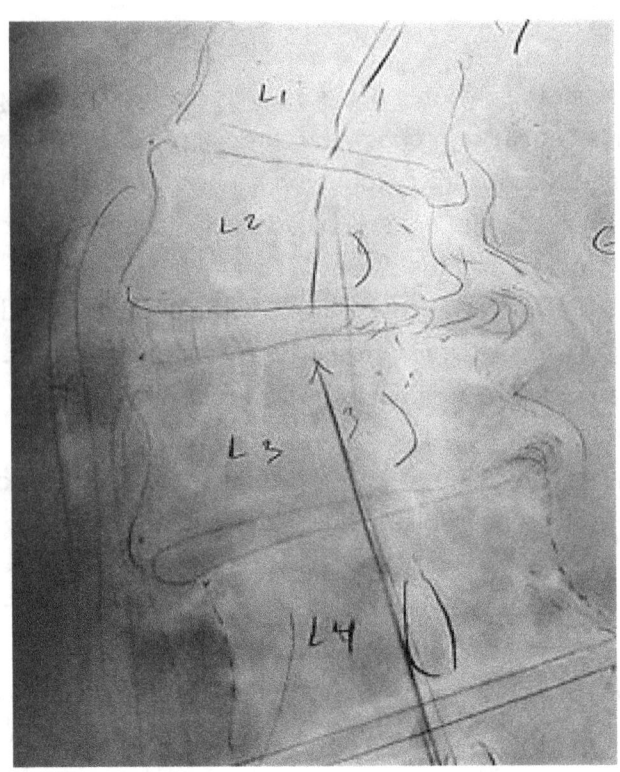
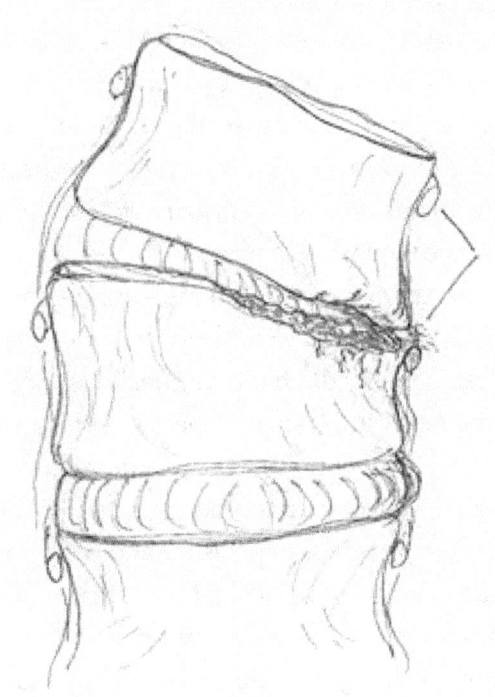

What continued my interest in Leo was the fact that sympathetic nerves from the lumbar vertebrae lead to the colon. Sympathetic nerve branches are located on both sides of the vertebrae near the top sides of the vertebral body. More particularly, nerves on the left side of the lumbar vertebrae go directly to the descending colon. In Leo's case, damage occurred to the left side of his lumbar vertebrae. His surgery involved removal of this section of the colon. His spinal injury matched perfectly to the section of his colon where cancer developed. As a young chiropractor, I was taught that nerve interference affected both the spinal nerves and the autonomic nerves to organs.

Leo's case filled me with a kind of scientific thrill — a feeling that I had glimpsed a biological truth about the physiology of a vertebral compression fracture and a bleeding spine. Since his case in 1985, I started asking for referral of cases where people had traumatic spinal fractures and then later ended with cancer or autoimmune disease. I was particularly interested in lateral compression fractures to the vertebral body. I continued tracking cases and discovered which injuries correlated with subsequent autoimmune diseases or cancers. Patterns emerged, and before long my theory gained credibility. At the time, studies were showing that nerves serve not only to conduct electrical signals throughout the body, but they also function to release proteins to the tissues. Studies on axon flow described microtubules within the nerve axon that allow small proteins to go down the nerves. I continued to push my idea: marrow stem cells are so small that they could penetrate damaged nerves and flow down the axon to an organ.

I wrote an article as a handout on my theory for patients, and their families and friends. I looked for patients with a history of spinal trauma that occurred before, but later led to; illness and cancer. Particularly I was looking for lateral compression fractures of the top end plates of vertebrae in the lumbar and thoracic regions. My theory gradually progressed with greater and greater detail, and my confidence grew that I had stumbled onto a valuable discovery. I began to chronicle injuries and subsequent maladies of other patients who worked on ranches or rode horses in their work. I found that spinal trauma typically preceded a person's autoimmune disease or cancer. Dozens of patient cases began to fall into place. Still I had no grasp of why injuries to the spine would bear any relation to cancer or of the disease. What was the mechanism? Do immune cells attack stem cells as foreign invaders? How long do the stem cells survive? In large numbers do the stem cells make genetic changes or mutation inside the local cells? I came up with more questions than answers.

To test my theory, I began to make assumptions about previous accidents even before viewing patients' x-rays. Frequently I would predict with a patient what level of spinal fracture they had. Some of these inquiries startled my patients, as they thought I had glimpsed their past almost as a mind reader. Though I'm not a research scientist, I often share with researchers my powerful curiosity about the etiology of disease. Because the practice of a small-town chiropractor involves regular contact with patients and their families, sometimes over many years, I was able to gather case histories that fit my theory. Not only did I want to help these folks live without pain, I wanted to help them heal whatever diseases they encountered. Since I came from a large family, and worked dozens of different jobs in my youth, I have been able to examine many compression fracture injuries to the spine.

Continued education for my chiropractic profession led me to studies on spinal disc damage. Other researchers have made observations that support my theory of spinal trauma and its link to illness. In the 1980s and 1990s, Japanese researchers associated herniated disc lesions with autoimmune diseases. Research just before the millennium blames various cancers on what scientists call "cancer stem cells." These studies support my theory of bleeding spine injuries and the link to cancer and autoimmune diseases I began collecting since the mid-1980s.

PROOF OF MY THEORY

On a late Monday night returning home with several copies of office magazines under my arm, I stepped through the door from the garage into my family room. A copy of the September 2003 issue of U.S. News & World Report fell onto my feet wide open to an article that verified my idea. I nearly flipped upside down and inside out! The story titled, "Seeds of Malignancy," by Nell Boyce, reported that top cancer research doctors discovered stem cells to present in 70% of cancer in the human body. They tagged them as cancer stem cells or CSCs. Yet the article related that science still did not know how the cancer stem cells arrived at the tissues. I called the cancer research doctors at MIT and Stanford. I explained to them how I believed stem cells found their way into the tissues. And they both said, "I'll have to think about that." I could have written that article.

NERVES PROVIDE HIGHWAYS FOR LEAKED STEM CELLS

Nothing fascinates a chiropractor more than the spine and its amazing ability to move and protect the spinal cord and nerves. Most chiropractic theories focus at the locations where nerve roots exit the spine. Two types of nerves branch off near the side of each vertebra: spinal nerves and sympathetic nerves. Spinal nerves travel to muscles and pain sensors. They control muscle tone and contraction and have pain receptor nerves that travel to skin and joint tissue. They register pain and help with balance, with the body's ability to sense balance and pressure, and to detect when damage or injury occurs. Another type of nerve located off the exiting pathway is the sympathetic nerve of the autonomic nervous system. The sympathetic nervous system helps the body react to danger: the fight or flight response where muscles leap into action and speed up certain organ systems, such as the heart rate, and slow down others, such as digestion. They also help maintain the homeostasis or wellness of organ tissues. Compare this to the nerves of the autonomic nervous system: parasympathetic nerves control automatic functions of a resting person, such as slowing the heart rate, urination, increase digestion and sexual arousal.

Sympathetic nerves end their pathways in the framework of organs and tissues. They exit out of the neck, thoracic and lumbar vertebrae. Leaked stem cells from damaged vertebrae may travel via these nerve pathways to their ends and enter the connective tissue of that organ. Since the stem cells arrive as undeveloped cells, they are treated as foreign virus-like substances and are attacked by the immune system. The initiation of autoimmune disease is complex and unknown. Since stem cells have genetic structure like that of the immune and tissue cells that attack them, the antibodies produced also attack normal cells. A nerve sending marrow stem cells into our tissues is like feeding cows their very own organs. The antibodies produced attack our own tissues.

Part of my training involved dissection of human cadavers to learn the body's structure in precise terms. Sympathetic nerves branch off the spinal nerve roots and immediately travel against and along the upper side portions of each vertebral body. The path of these nerves lies so close to the bone that leaked stem cells have quick and easy absorption into their lining or sympathetic ganglia. Most compression injuries occur to the superior plate of the vertebral body. It's somewhat like smashing down the top of a cardboard box. With one sharp blow a vertebra suddenly opens a crack or is compressed down like stepping on the top of a block of Styrofoam. Rarely does the interior or bottom plate suffer damage unless it's a severe compression fracture.

Most people think bones are rigid structures. Actually, bones are quite compressible and flexible, normally rebounding to their original shape. Vertebral end plates, due to their structure, flex enough during accidents to escape serious injury in most cases. While the outside structure is more rigid, the central portion of the top of the end plate resembles a trampoline — yielding, rebounding and resilient. But after a compression injury, end plates are crushed. They tend to split or tear. The disc itself may split and allow seepage of stem cells from the red marrow.

Injuries to the middle of the end plates during puberty, and during the growth hormone years, heal quickly as a cartilage node. In a child, cartilage nodes may form from herniated discs that protrude into the vertebral endplates. These nodes are known as Schmorl's nodes. Considerable research now focuses on the end plates of vertebrae, and how damaged end plates may trigger disease. During the repair process, end-plate mineralization occurs and reduces exchange of fluids and nutrients from the marrow to the disc. This resulting calcification can lead to further degeneration of the disc and joints. The vertebral end plates are injured in a variety of ways. They can be compressed, crushed, split, torn, or separated from the intervertebral disc.

Stem cells — tiny protein seeds containing inaugural DNA — may act as antigens or foreign molecules when they are immature and escape their container in bone marrow. Is it possible they can flow down nerve axons almost like roadways into connective tissues of organs? Only further research on my theory will determine whether this theory is correct. The immune system may react to undeveloped stem cells the way it would an invading virus or bacterium. The immune system forms antibodies to attack loose stem cells, thereby initiating autoimmune disease. If one kidney falls to autoimmune disease, often the malady migrates to the other kidney because it shares the same type of connective tissue. To fight antigenic stem cells, the immune system also devours nearby connective tissue resulting in inflammation and loss of essential support tissues.

Science has found the greater number of proportion of cancer stem cells, CSCs, within the cancer tissue the greater the aggressiveness of the cancer and the difficulty in complete eradication of the cancer.

The attacking immune system appears to thrive on connective tissue made of collagen, attracted to the stem cells that penetrate the tissue. Eventually, the thinning of connective tissue causes weakened structure, dilated tissues, and diminished function. For example, a polyp in the colon results from dilatation and swelling of the wall of the organ. The dilating or expansion of an abdominal aneurysm occurs from an immune attack. In most diseases it is the loss of connective or interstitial tissue of the organ that causes the organ to fail. The connective tissue is made of collagen. Specialized non-dividing cells of the organ — muscle, brain, heart, or kidney — rarely are the ones taken over by the immune system. An organ's connective tissue system fails after being attacked by the immune system, and the resulting progression of organ disease can be slow or quick depending on healing and risk factors of the individual. An organ cannot continue to function without its essential structure.

Given the strong similarities between tumor-initiating cells and stem cells, researchers have found CSCs do arise both from stem cells and adult differentiated cells with different malignancies.

It has long been proposed that cancer and tumors form and proliferate from the actions of a small population of unique cells. In my theory of bleeding spine injuries, the degree of inflammation correlates to how each person's immune system handles the entry of stem cells into an organ's tissue. Poor supporting response and high concentration of stem cells in the tissue may lead quickly to serious disease such as cancer. A good immune response to marrow stem cells with a strong antibody vaccinating type reaction may lead to chronic conditions such as Crohn's disease. The initial entrance of stem cells may set up the tissues for a long illness when antibodies are formed against local cells.

Illnesses are site-specific, correlating directly to stem cell presence. Some cancer stem cells, possibly disarmed by the immune system, lie dormant in connective tissues. Where cancer develops, in most cases autoimmune disease may have preceded the cancer. When the immune system overreacts, or cannot handle leaked stem cells in the region, it loses control and a seed of malignancy can occur. A genetic mutation occurs within host cells. The self-renewal genetic factors overtake the cells and proliferation is rampant. Other immune suppressant factors may degrade the body's ability to ward off serious disease, such as exposure to environmental toxins, medications, and pollutants. People who were not colostrum-fed or had poor nutrition, and other habits that effect immune system efficiency, will fall more easily into disease.

There are three components to an autoimmune disease development. Stem cells, immune cells and the base tissue collagen cells are all a part of the mix. Stem cells presence in the collagen structure of an organ tissue provokes an immune response. The renewal process of the base collagen may increase or decrease with the presence of stem cells. The immune response can control the inflammatory action if the stem cell numbers are small, and the immune system is healthy and not compromised. Up to 70% of a person's immune system may not be present if that person was not colostrum fed right at birth.

Once the body's immune system forms antibodies against leaked stem cells, those antibodies are coded for permanent production. Antibodies are produced within a specific collagen tissue of an organ. If stem cells enter the bladder connective tissues, antibodies will be developed targeting bladder collagen. If the stem cells enter the colon, the colon comes under immune attack and antibodies will be produced that inflame and damage colon tissue. If the ovaries or uterus have a stem cell activated immune response in women, antibodies will be produced against those organs and make them susceptible to disease or failure.

There are three components to an autoimmune disease development. Stem cells, immune cells and the base tissue collagen cells are all a part of the mix. Stem cells presence in the collagen structure of an organ tissue provokes an immune response. The renewal process of the base collagen may increase or decrease with the presence of stem cells. The immune response can control the inflammatory action if the stem cell numbers are small, and the immune system is healthy and not compromised.

Each organ's connective tissue is different. Therefore, autoimmunity is specific to that organ's or tissue's collagen framework. Stem cells may leak from fractures of a vertebra or rib. A herniated intervertebral disc has been shown to lead to autoimmune disease. A lateral compression fracture allows stem cells to penetrate damaged sympathetic nerves or ganglion which channel to various pathways to individual organs. Sometimes an auto-antibody is produced against a broad range of collagen or connective tissue of multiple organs. An anterior compression fracture can make stem cells leak into the thoracic or abdominal cavity, and produce disease in multiple organs, or cause systemic lupus. An arch fracture of a vertebra can cause melanoma to the skin or multiple sclerosis within the spinal cord.

With proper care and nutrition, the body is amazing in its healing ability. There might be inflammation and autoimmune disease for awhile, but a healthy body bounces back after repairing tissue damage from bleeding stem cells. In later chapters I will give examples of a variety of illnesses and cancers that I believe were initiated by stem cell leakage. I will also give encouragement by providing nutritional advice that may promote a better immune and healing response. I wish I could prevent injury for all humans, but gravity has its presence. There will always be injuries. A strong and vital immune system will be the answer to removing cancer stem cells. As genetic research develops more sophistication, soon our immune system will be guided by human-modified stem cells that can be used to destroy previously leaked stem cells.

CHAPTER 3

Vertebral Compression Fracture

• • •

JANE'S STORY IN THE LOCAL paper brings light to the debilitating effect medications have on our spine. She is a renowned architect known for her unique style for over thirty years. Jane can be seen around town in a well decorated scooter she has been using since a collapsed spine two years ago. Having problems as a child with her lungs, she was told her breathing problems were due to asthma.

Two years ago, Jane began feeling increased pain in her upper back. Eventually she was diagnosed with a severe compression fracture in her thoracic vertebrae. Years of steroid medications for her asthma had destroyed her bone density. Doctors attempted back surgery however the unstable vertebrae had continued to affect her nerve cord and weakened her legs. Her spirit undaunted, Jane fashioned her living room into a workplace to avoid the upstairs, while she gained back some strength in her legs.

Count the segments of the human spine and you'll find it consists of 33 vertebrae that extend from the base of the head to the pelvis. The vertebrae are stacked in a vertical column and directly fastened together by soft hydrated intervertebral discs at the front and a pair of facets or joints at the back half of the column. The spinal column houses the spinal cord and exiting nerves in a way that allows flexibility and movement. Fluid discs, back muscles, ligaments, and tendons provide spinal motion and stability.

The spinal column serves to protect the spinal cord and 31 pairs of nerve roots that branch off the spine. The spine provides stability and support for the head, chest, and shoulders, allowing the body to stand and walk upright. The spine enables flexibility and mobility of the upper body. Adjacent vertebrae are held together by a fluid fibrous disc that serves as a shock absorber by cushioning the stress forces placed on the spine when someone walks, runs, or jumps. The intervertebral discs contain about 80 percent water and account for a third of the spine's length. Joints called facets also contain cartilage and a large amount of water.

Each vertebra has a front pressurized box-like structure called the vertebral body that consists of firm calcified bone on the outside and soft fiber fluid matrix of germinating red bone marrow on the inside. The vertebral body has its own internal fluid pressure due to blood supply and fluid exchange. The internal matrix of red bone marrow contains stem cells of hematopoietic system which produces millions of red blood cells, platelets, and white blood cells by the minute. The red marrow contains cells that are in a multitude of levels of maturity. There are several histological stages that red marrow cells must grow through to become an adult cell and be released into the blood circulation. The red marrow does not release immature cells and the very bone that protects it, secures this process. Inaugural stem cells are somatically stored and capped off for storage by the end plates, or top and bottom connective tissue plates that join to the intervertebral disc.

Scientists say there is unequivocal proof that stem cells exist in the hematopoietic system of the red marrow and has led to the discovery and isolation of many tissue-specific stem and progenitor cells.

The vertebral end plates guard the red marrow and feed nutrients in and out the intervertebral disc. Water, proteins, and nutrients flow into the disc more from a pressure gradient than direct blood flow. The vertebral end plate is the top and bottom of the vertebral body and grows in thickness during puberty years to add height to each segment. Proper growth plate development gives us our normal height at the end of our growth cycle.

Joints of the body and spine are very healthy when puberty and the growth period take place. Production of growth hormone and protein factors signal blood vessel growth and fabulous circulation to the growing ends of bones. It just so happens the joints of our body are adjacent to this great vascular change. When production of growth hormone slows at the end of puberty, blood supply to the endplate and intervertebral disc ceases. From this time on there is no direct blood supply to any of your joints in the body. It is very important to maintain active motion between the vertebrae and all joints of the body to keep nutrients and water flowing in and out of the disc and other joints. Adult spines need to be constantly in proper motion.

To maintain a healthy intervertebral disc and vertebral end plate, there must be constant proper motion between the vertebral segments. Non-movement means deterioration. Move it or lose it! Once puberty is finished in your early twenties the blood supply to growing cartilage ceases. When you simply move a finger or knee joint after puberty, the surrounding ligament tissue called the capsule causes suction or vacuum of pressure to draw nutrients into our collagen-based cartilage. Put a splint on a joint and immobilize it, and within twenty-four hours you start losing collagen cells. Death to our joints if we don't move them!

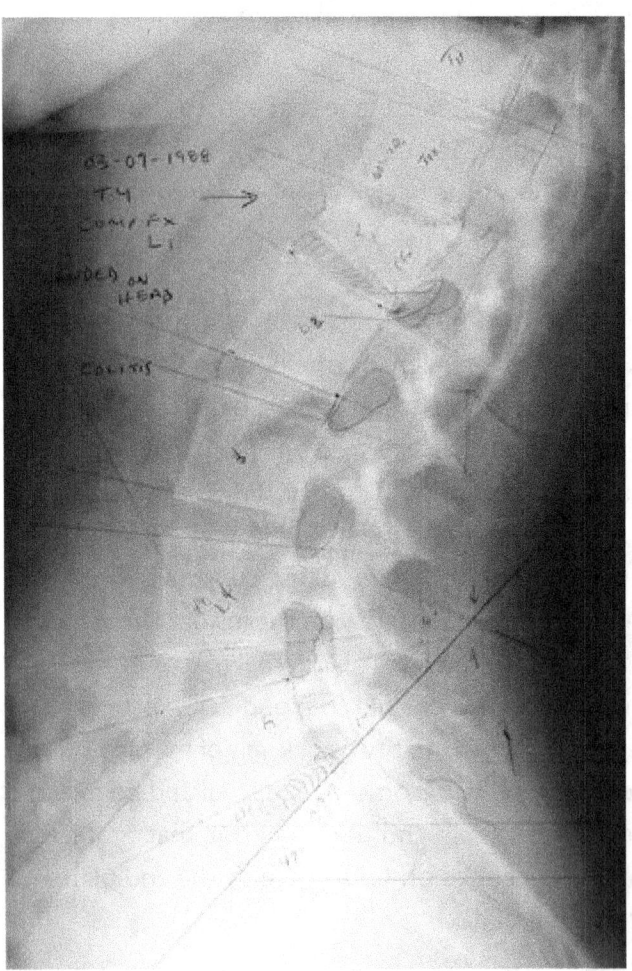

At the back of the vertebral body sits an arch of bone called the posterior arch. The posterior part of the vertebra contains red bone marrow as does its anterior part, the vertebral body. The arch has two surfaces for the facet joints and creates a spinal canal or tunnel that houses and protects the pathway for the spinal cord. The spinal cord originates at the base of the brain and ends at the first lumbar vertebra. The end of the spinal cord separates into nerve bundles known as the cauda equina or horse's tail.

The vertebral body of a healthy spine is like a suitcase that is compressible and flexible. It can withstand compressive forces and is malleable. It has some resiliency and can bounce back to its original shape after momentary minor compression. The vertebral body can stand considerable pressure but when the compressive force applied exceeds the load limit of the bone, one or more vertebrae can collapse. With a compression fracture, the box-like body of the vertebra cracks or collapses, somewhat like stepping on a block of Styrofoam. The resulting fracture produces a dent in the box, a change in the shape of the vertebral body, and creates a loss of height between vertebral segments.

Vertebral compression fractures change the shape and function of both the outer shell of the vertebral body, known as the cortical bone, and the inner marrow bone, known as cancellous bone. Compression fractures can occur at any level of the vertebrae but happen most commonly in the lower thoracic and upper lumbar vertebrae. It can result in a mild dent in the end plate to a moderate deformity of the spine. These fractures occur as the result of traumatic car accidents, falls from height, or from everyday activities such as rising from a chair if osteoporosis or degenerative bone damage is present. Osteoporotic spinal fractures are unusual in that they may occur without apparent trauma.

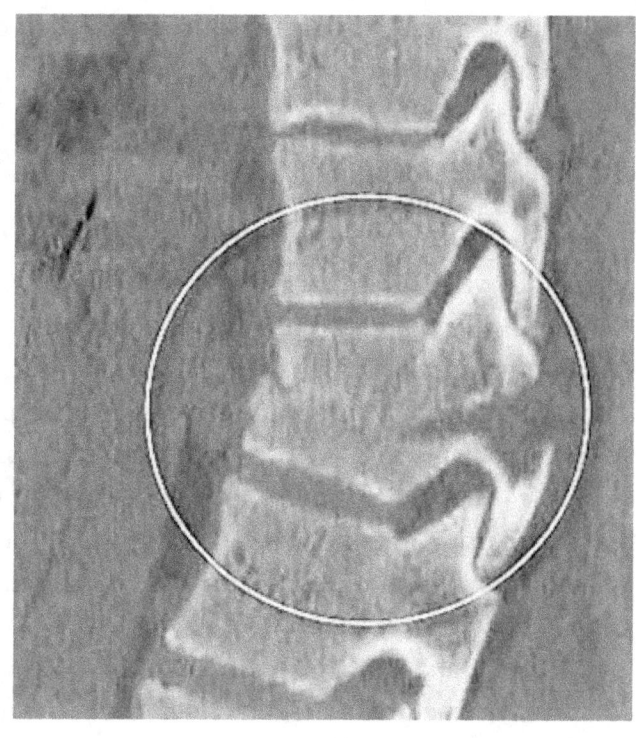

Vertebral compression fractures range from large burst fractures with pain, to small compression fractures with no pain, and fractures due to osteoporosis and pre-weakened bone. There are varying types of vertebral fractures. One type is a wedge fracture, which receives its name from a collapse of the anterior or posterior of the vertebral body.

Another type of fracture is a biconcave or mid-plate fracture. This involves a collapse of the central portion of one or both vertebral body end plates. A crush fracture is a severe collapse of the entire vertebral body. Lateral or side fracture is a top side compression to one side, right or left of the vertebra. Lateral compression fractures are produced when extreme lateral flexion of the spine occurs.

Wedge fractures are the most common fractures and occur most frequently at the mid-thoracic and upper lumbar regions in both men and women. Crush fractures also have a higher tendency to occur in the mid- to lower-thoracic vertebrae, and not the lumbar region. Unlike other types of fractures, biconcave fractures are equally as likely to occur in lower lumbar vertebrae as in other spinal levels. Dislocation fractures of the spine occur in accidents that pull the segments of the spine apart. They are known as chance fractures. Chance fractures are also known as seatbelt fractures. They are hyper-flexion distraction injuries where the vertebrae are forced apart from one another. They are primarily due to the installation of lap belts and shoulder belts in automobiles. There are two types of chance fractures: bony chance, and ligamentous chance. Bony chance fracture is severe; the vertebra is fractured and pulled apart completely across the middle of the entire vertebra. Ligamentous chance fracture is a separation of the vertebra at its end plate from the intervertebral disc, like pulling the lid from a sealed container. These fractures are difficult to image as the endplate and body seal back together after some contents have leaked out.

Non-traumatic fractures of the vertebral body also occur from two causes. Osteoporotic fractures happen when the bone of the vertebral body is thin and weak. Stepping hard down a step or rising from a chair may collapse a weak vertebra. The most common cause of contemporary osteoporotic fracture is the use of blood thinning medication. Avascular necrosis compression fractures can occur during the bone growth years. Vertebral end plates injured by mild compression injury or fracture can lead to acute avascular necrosis to the growing plates of the vertebrae. Damaged vascularization can destroy bone growth, and further collapse of the vertebra can occur. In the early stages of end plate growth, the loss of one side of the blood supply leads to a laterally wedge-shaped vertebral body, and scoliosis. Scoliosis — lateral curvature of the spine — and kyphosis — reversed curve or hunchback spine — will be explained in the next chapter.

Vertebral compression fractures have physical, psychological, and social consequences, and are associated with increased mortality. The physical consequences of vertebral compression fractures include back pain, scoliosis, kyphosis, spinal deformity, decreased lung capacity and pulmonary function, impaired physical function, sleeping problems, and loss of appetite. Observed psychological consequences include anxiety, depression, loss of self-esteem, frustration and feeling of defeat. In this book, I will offer a theory of physiology where vertebral compression fractures bleed out stem cells. The undeveloped molecules enter nearby tissues causing local inflammation or provoke distal attacks by the immune system as they enter an organ's connective tissue via the sympathetic nerve pathway.

X-ray, CT, and MRI imaging have been underutilized in studying the location and physiology of vertebral compression fractures. These fractures can be identified by loss of structure, edema, or fluid clefts within the vertebral body. Medical studies give little attention to compression fractures and other spinal structures, such as vertebral implant outcomes, acute vertebral disc injury, and posterior elements, including arch and facet joints, spinal ligaments, and paraspinal musculature. In some studies of vertebral compression fracture, images showed a high incidence of end plate injury along with vertebral disc injury. Of a hundred cases of vertebral compression fracture, anterior or superior vertebral end plate injury accounted for 39 percent. Inferior end plate injury accounted for 12 percent. Injury to both ends of the vertebra was observed in 29 percent of the levels. The pattern of intervertebral disc injury was similar, with injury to the disk above the fracture in 36 percent of the cases.

Conclusions: vertebral end plate injury is commonly seen in traumatic and osteoporotic vertebral compression fractures. Furthermore, this type of damage is frequently associated with injury to the adjacent intervertebral disc. These findings are often underreported but should be described because they may have important implications for symptomatic presentation, patient management, and outcomes.

Evidence of cracked vertebrae and vertebral compression fractures is increasing steadily along with the increase in human longevity. Presently, vertebral compression fractures affect nearly 25 percent of all postmenopausal women and 40 percent of women aged 80 and older. Anyone with significant back pain, especially women over 50, should see a physician. One or more symptoms can indicate that you may be suffering from acute vertebral compression fracture, burst fracture, or cracked vertebrae. In patients with these conditions, sitting leads to severe back pain. Standing or walking worsens back pain. Lying down provides only minor back pain relief. Bending and twisting is difficult and painful to perform. A loss of height may occur as the spine becomes deformed or curved, taking on a hunchback shape.

The main causes of vertebral compression fractures are trauma and osteoporosis. Osteoporosis affects more than 10 million elderly Americans. Of those affected, 80 percent are female. It is estimated that as many as 14 million Americans will have osteoporosis by 2020 if efforts are not made to control the disease. Osteoporosis, which weakens bone over time, results in more than 1.5 million fragility fractures annually in the U.S., of which

900,000 are spine fractures. The most common cause of compressive spinal fractures is medication-induced osteoporosis. Most oral medication destroys and weakens the liver output of essential tissue-building proteins. In 2011, studies were released that Fosamax and Boniva may weaken bone structure and cause fractures. The very medications promoted for bone formation ended up causing bone loss and fracture! In the U.S. alone, it is estimated that this bone weakening metabolic disease is the cause of 750,000 to 800,000 vertebral compression fractures annually. This mainly effects the population with poor diet and overly medicated.

Vertebral compression fractures can be very painful and can have impact on the spinal cord or nerve roots of the individual. A severe posterior fracture near the front of the spinal cord can lead to paralysis of the muscle system. A milder fracture can be due to medications that thin the blood or have an ill effect on the liver. The liver produces and releases tens of thousands of protein strands into the bloodstream every millisecond. Liver protein production and release is extremely important to maintain bone stability. Sometimes bone loss fractures are clinically silent and are also known as silent or spontaneous fractures. They may occur at several levels of the spine. This means the individual experiences little or no discomfort. In older patients, pain is often attributed to the natural aging process, and tolerated by the individual without seeking medical evaluation.

Symptoms of a compression fracture other than pain include loss of body height, pain when standing or walking, evidence of kyphosis, dowager's hump, or humpback at the top of the back, which is common in older women. Loss of balance, psychological disturbances, or neurological symptoms, such as numbness and tingling, also may occur. These symptoms are serious, but if my theory is true, that stem cells flow out of vertebral fractures into tissues and nerves, then more serious disease such as autoimmune disease and cancer can develop quickly or over a prolonged period.

CHAPTER 4

Stem Cell: Creator, Culprit, and Cure

● ● ●

A STEM CELL IS THE smallest genetic molecule or protein strand coded DNA which can renew itself called self-renewal and it can produce sets of different cells through a process called differentiation. The inaugural stem cell is undifferentiated - not a true cell but a blueprint for cells. In the embryonic state, stem cells start out very early and control the development and production of all 216 specialized cells in the body. Embryonic stem cells are the creator of various tissues and organs, including highly specialized future non-dividing cells of heart, brain, muscle, and liver tissue. The base stem cells that are unspecialized and reproducing themselves only are called adult stem cells. When inaugural stem cells reproduce, they always make one exact copy of themselves indefinitely. This allows them to not only increase their own numbers but make a cell that goes on to increase the cell growth of other tissues. The specialized cells of the brain, heart and muscle are produced only in the beginning embryonic stage. Each person is given a certain number, and normally no more will be produced.

Adult stem cells - these are not as versatile for research purposes because they are specific to certain cell types, such as blood, intestines, skin, and muscle. The term "adult stem cell" may be misleading because both children and adults have them. Adult stem cells are just a stage away from embryonic stem cells, and scientists have learned to de-program adult stem cells back to pluripotent embryonic cells. They are also known as marrow stem cells, or somatic stem cells. Adult stem cells have been found in many more tissues. However, the majority are found in the marrow of the spinal system. They reside in the skull, vertebrae, ribs, and pelvis. One group of adult stem cells is known as hematopoietic stem cells. They are responsible for forming all the blood cells in the body. A second group called stromal, or mesenchymal, stem cells are non-blood-forming, but instead help generate and heal bone, cartilage, fat, and all connective tissues that develop and support organs and tissue systems.

Research on stem cells has been active for more than sixty years. Most research started on adult stem cells from the bone marrow. Scientists seek to reproduce stem cells into specialized cells to help repair our damaged and aging bodies. There are many areas in medicine in which stem cell research could have a significant impact. For example, there are a variety of diseases and injuries in which a patient's cells or tissues are destroyed and could be replaced by tissue or organ transplants. Stem cells may be able to generate new tissue in these cases, and even cure diseases for which there currently is no adequate therapy. Diseases and injuries that could see revolutionary advances include Alzheimer's and Parkinson's disease, diabetes, spinal cord injury, heart disease, stroke, arthritis, cancer, burns and skin maladies. Stem cells must be modified correctly for therapy use.

Cancer researchers announced in 2003 that stem cells from bone marrow are responsible for the repeating cell division of cancer. Stem cells are now known to be involved in all cancers and illnesses of the body. Scientists are trying hard to find out how these small molecules of DNA are so wonderful on one side of human physiology yet can be so dark and disruptive on the other. Understanding the codes of stem cells will help scientists make gains in preventing birth defects and cancer. When the genetic basis for cell development is understood better, stem cells may be altered to help prevent and cure disease.

Stem cells of the hematopoietic system of red bone marrow are capped off and contained in the axial spine. This includes retainment in the vertebrae, ribs, cranium, sacrum, and pelvis. Stem cells do not belong outside of these marrow cavities unless they have differentiated or grown in stages to become complete cells. They mature, develop, or differentiate into a particular cell, such as a red blood cell, white blood cell or platelet.

Cancer stem cells are formed many ways. The three ways below include epigenetic changes to stem cells, progenitor cells and differentiated cells.

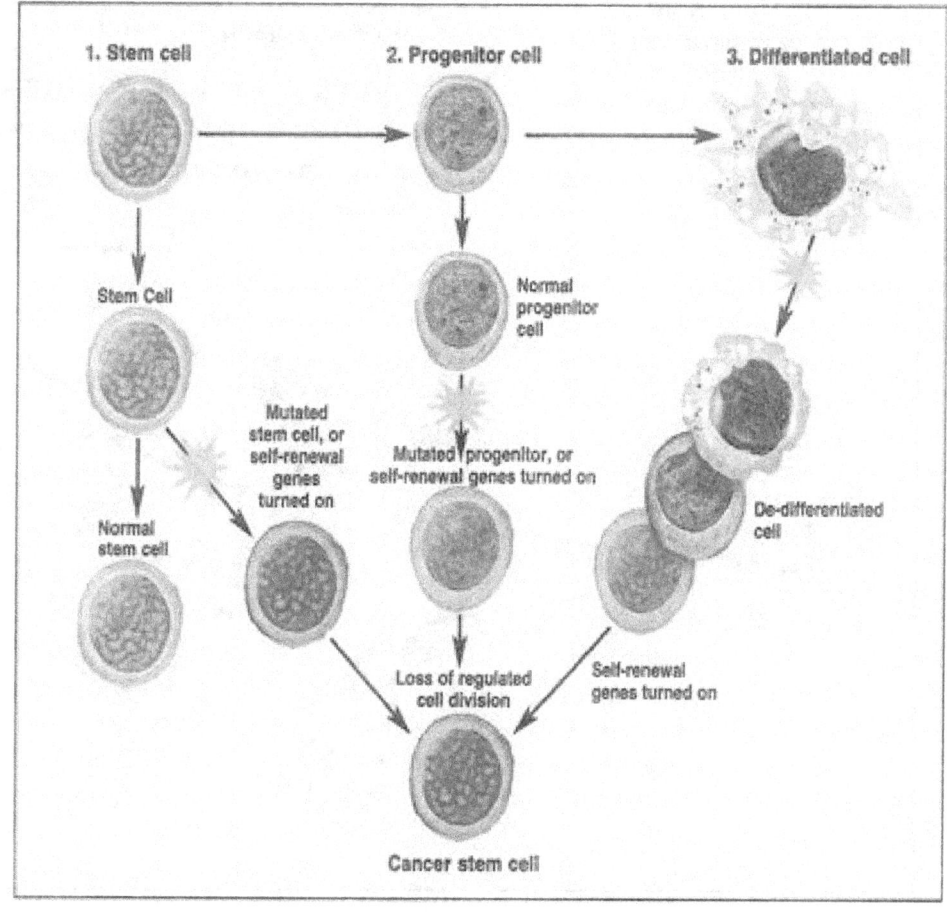

Some cells when they first develop become too large to escape out of the blood supply, but they mature to a smaller size and then travel on their way. During a compression fracture of the spine, however, under-developed stem cells are forced out of their environment, and flow like tiny grains of sand into tissues and vessels. The immune system reacts to leaked stem cells as if they were viruses.

Stem cells that leak out of from injured vertebrae are usually removed by the immune system that is present in local tissues and circulation. Lymphatic channels and lymph nodes are strategically positioned along each side of the spine to combat injury and stem cell bleeding. Branches of the sympathetic nerves are located alongside the upper vertebral body. These nerve pathways are right where a compression fracture occurs. So closely positioned that after trauma to the marrow and nerve, penetration, and absorption of raw antigenic stem like molecules can occur. Immune cells, originally created by stem cells, do not recognize their creators, and begin attacking and devouring the invading stem cells. If stem cells enter local tissue in large numbers, they may overwhelm the immune system response and end up converting and mutating local cells.

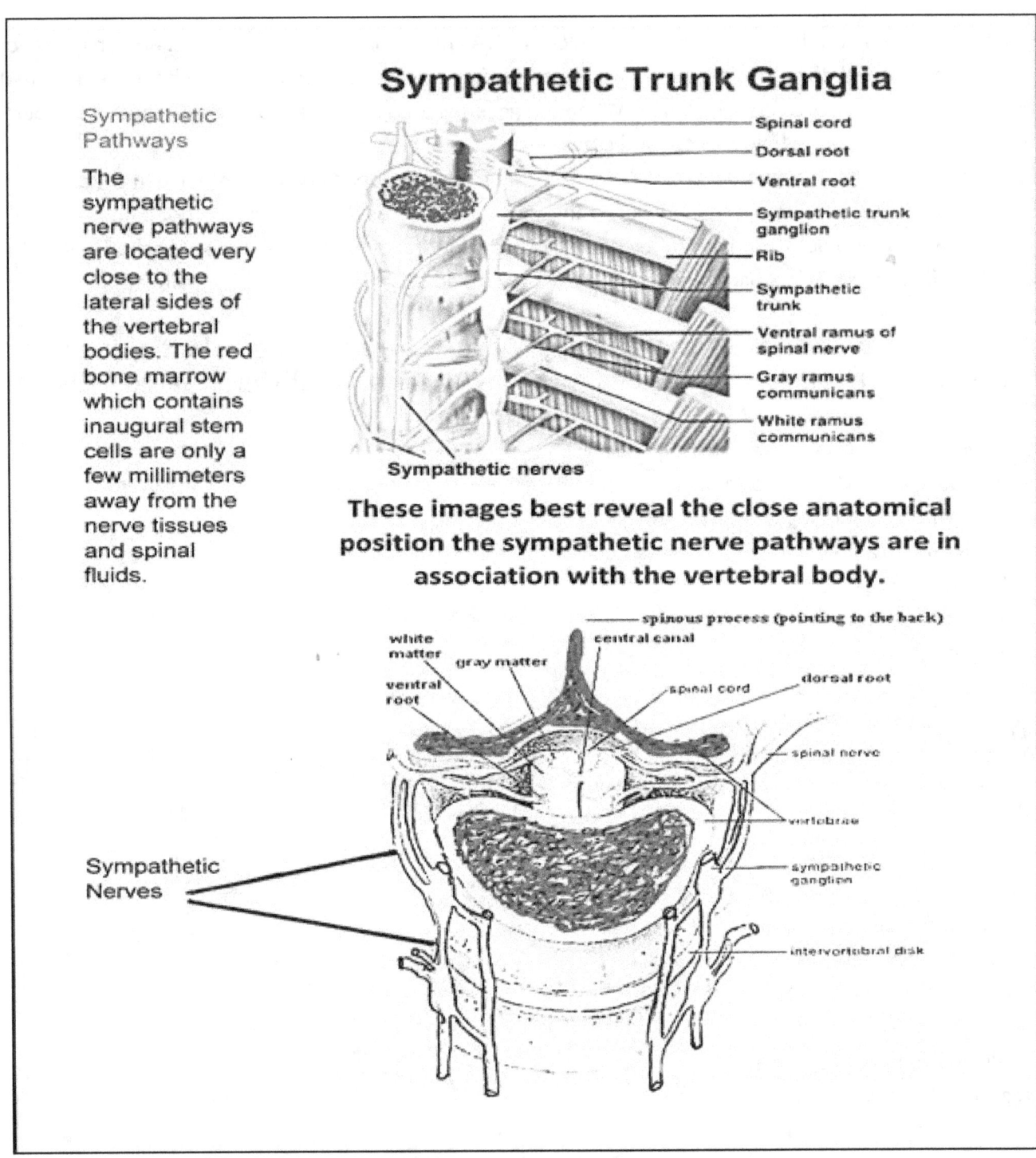

Sympathetic Pathways

The sympathetic nerve pathways are located very close to the lateral sides of the vertebral bodies. The red bone marrow which contains inaugural stem cells are only a few millimeters away from the nerve tissues and spinal fluids.

These images best reveal the close anatomical position the sympathetic nerve pathways are in association with the vertebral body.

Stem cells of the red bone marrow are so small they can penetrate nearly any tissue, including damaged nerve, vessel, and spinal cord linings. They can inflame local nerves and flow down the microtubules of the axons of the sympathetic nerves. Once inside the nerve axon, stem cells go freely, and escape attack from immune cells until they reach the end of the nerve. When large concentrations of stem cells enter the connective tissue of an organ or tissue system, a catastrophic immune response will develop.

Bleeding of Stem Cells

After impact to the cancellous bone of the vertebral body, the damaged red bone marrow bleeds and flows out into nerve tissue, spinal fluid flow or into the body cavity. The hematopoietic system or red bone marrow contains inaugural stem cells. The bleeding flow can contain stem cells or parts of their genetic DNA. The healing process activates the immune system and blood into a cellular battle. Yet the matrix of the red bone marrow is full of immature red blood and white blood cells. A fracture to the axial spine includes damage to the red bone marrow cellular matrix. A fracture of the long bones involves yellow or fat contained marrow. I believe damage to the red bone marrow matrix creates a volatile healing process due to the many histological levels of cells it contains. Are platelets in place to seal off the crushed bone? Does the impact to the red marrow damage the stem cells to produce an epigenetic flow of DNA into the nearby nerves and circulation systems? Are some stem cells taken up by the immune system and completely or partly deactivated? Do damaged stem cell particles lay dormant and then arise later to seed a malignancy?

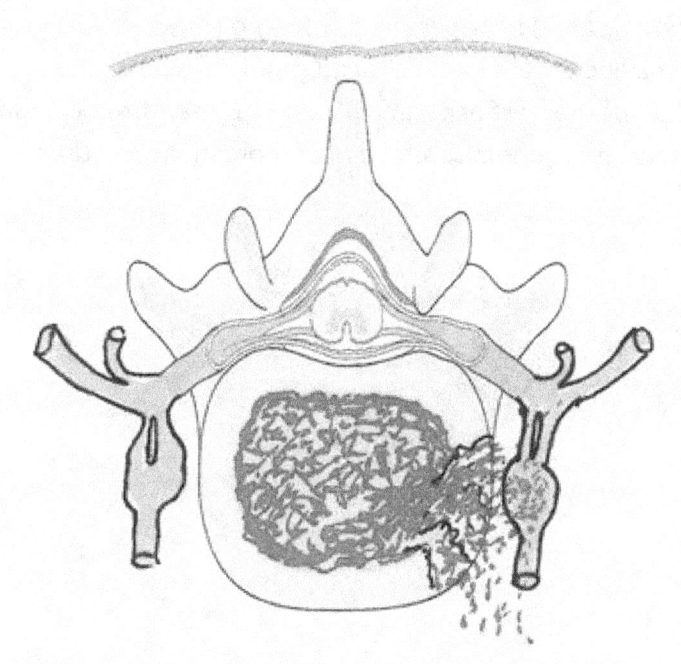

Stem cells are small enough to penetrate nerves and also the meningeal covering of the spinal cord and enter the spinal fluid flow. The compression injury can weaken nerve and spinal coverings allowing uptake of cellular debris.

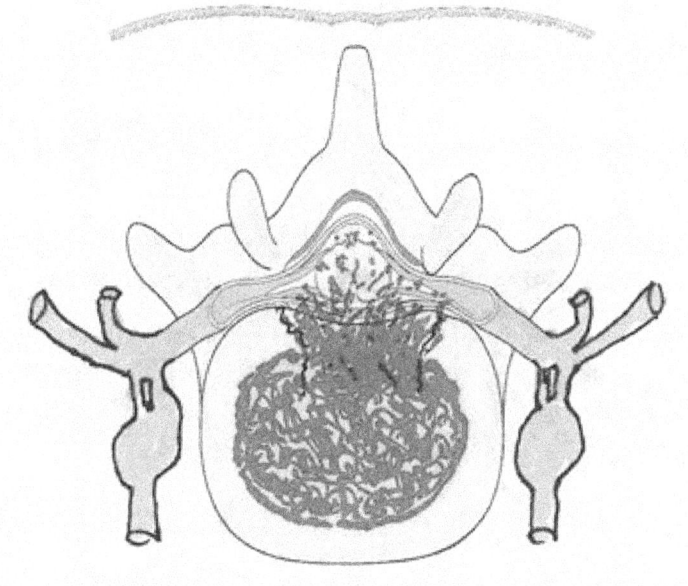

Once red marrow stem cells exit the sympathetic nerves into connective tissue sections of the colon or other organs, immune cells attack them. Local blood supply of the tissues may allow the stem cells to rapidly reproduce themselves. The reaction of the immune system becomes desperate and violent. Tissue destruction can occur so rapidly that the body is literally eating itself. This is known as a catastrophic immune response. After a simple traumatic accident, a person may feel no illness, yet the groundwork for many problems may be initiated. Stem cells may penetrate local cells and produce genetic changes to preserve themselves. Thousands of these cells can prompt the start of a tumor. Stem cells may flow down into several branches of autonomic nerves and cause antigenic reactions in several different organs at one time.

CHAPTER 5

Scoliosis and Kyphosis

● ● ●

A MAJOR PORTION OF MY research for this book involves searching for, examining, and treating, spinal injuries that crush or crack the vertebral body on the top lateral edge on one side, right or left. Typically, a lateral compression fracture to the vertebral body involves one vertebra tipping over and pushing down forcibly into the vertebra below on one side. The lateral force can cause a compression fracture to the side of the vertebral body and damage or herniate the intervertebral disc This creates a lateral curvature the spine — known as spinal scoliosis. Lateral compression injuries to the spine develop a lateral curve or scoliosis by three mechanisms. One involves direct lateral bone height loss, a second involves a lateral tear or herniation to the intervertebral disc. The scoliosis mechanisms can occur together or separately depending on the intensity of the trauma. A third cause of scoliosis occurs during the bone growing years, where a lateral trauma disrupts the upper lateral half of the blood supply to the growing end plate, stopping the normal growth of the vertebral body on that side.

The tilted shape of one vertebral body, or a lateral disc injury, allows the vertebra above to tip over to one side. Compression or disc injuries in hyper flexion or extreme side bending lead to thoracic or lumbar scoliosis. Compression fractures to an adult's vertebral body heal more slowly and less effectively than similar injuries in a child. Mild injuries in children can lead to scoliosis when the blood supply to growing end plate of the vertebral body is crushed with a side-bending spinal injury. The blood circulation for vertebra's plate growth discontinues or fails to match the other side of the vertebral body and produces a permanent lateral curvature to the spine.

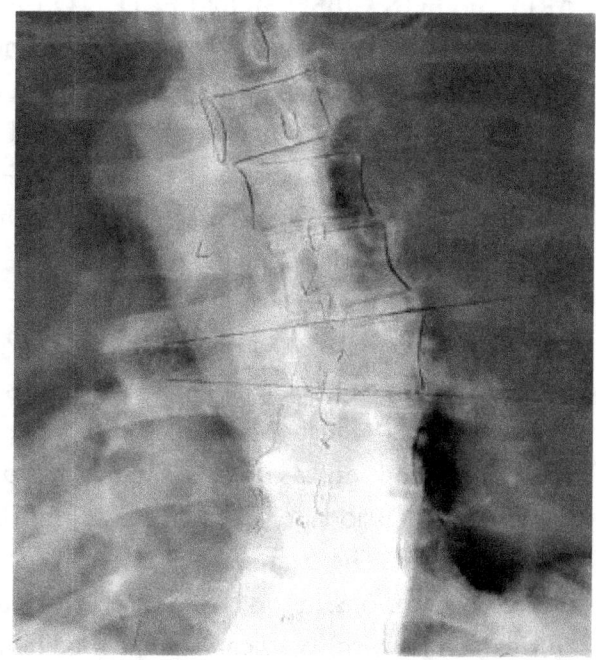

An injury that flexes the upper body violently forward tends to compress the front half of the vertebral body. This is known as an anterior compression fracture. This type of fracture causes a downward slope to the top front half of the vertebral body and allows the vertebra above to tip forward over the injured vertebra below. An anterior compression injury also crushes down the front half of the intervertebral disc. The front portion of the intervertebral disc can split on the inside and herniate without fracture. This also allows the forward tilting of the normal vertebra above the injury. The appearance of the posture is then rounded backward, a condition

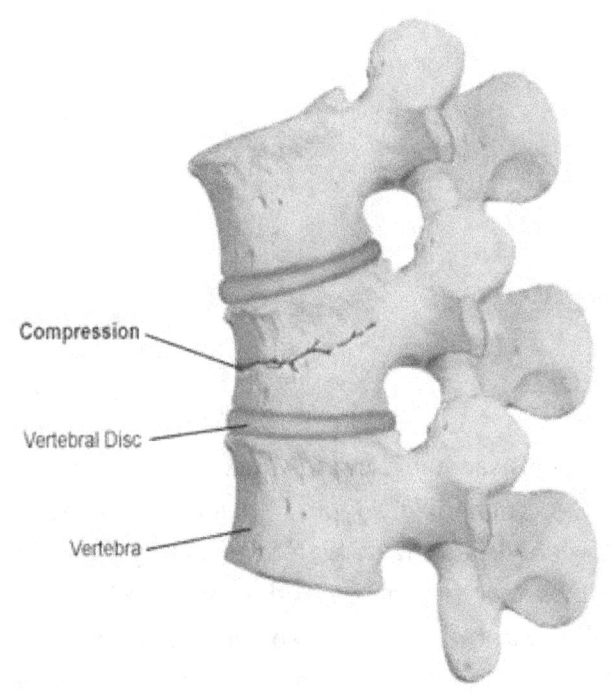

known as kyphosis that mostly plagues adults. Viewing such a person's spine from the side, the upper or lower back protrudes backward as a reverse curved spine. It appears as a hunchback or slouched posture.

A healthy spine has a slight natural curve when looking from the side. This natural curve has a normal range, and the usual spinal curvature helps humans move forward gracefully and absorb shocks. When spinal trauma accentuates the curvature into an abnormal range, scoliosis or kyphosis can cause back pain, instability of posture, uneven hips or shoulders, or a spine that deteriorates into osteoarthritis, also known as degenerative joint disease. Kyphosis in adults can be caused by forward trauma to the spine. When bone weakness is present, such as osteoporosis, kyphosis can result from even mild activity such as rising from a chair. Osteoporosis may be a common cause of anterior vertebral fractures. My studies have largely been of trauma-induced fracture, although I will comment in another chapter about spontaneous vertebral fractures. Medications, hormonal imbalances, and poor diet or digestive problems can lead to such weakening of the bone structure that even standing up puts enough stress to cause a spontaneous compression fracture. Prior compression fractures along with medications that thin the blood can easily lead to silent or spontaneous vertebral compression fractures.

Early Sports Obsession Leads to Neck Injury

Early in my practice a ten-year-old boy named Andrew came into my office complaining of neck and upper back pain with restriction of neck movement. He had difficulty holding his head up. X-rays revealed that all his neck and upper back vertebrae had irregularly shaped top and bottom end plates. It looked as if he had been bouncing on his head, crushing his cervical and thoracic vertebrae one into the other. His vertebral endplates gave an appearance known as Scheuermann's disease. The vertebral plates looked as if they had been punched in and roughened by multiple traumas.

This was serious because vertebrae injury before or during the growing years may impair complete and normal bone height. I asked him about his background, especially his participation in sports. Sure enough, he was an avid soccer player. More interestingly, his style of playing soccer involved leaping into the air and using his head to pass the ball or bounce it into the opposing team's goal zone. This move is not only legal in soccer; it is especially common as players gain skill and power. He was obsessed with heading the soccer ball, especially in practice! Professional soccer players can move the ball down the field with graceful arcs from one player's head to the next. The strategy may help win soccer games, but the spine loses. The brain may also suffer slight repeated concussions. In this child's case, I advised him to refrain from further compression to his head and neck and treated him with spinal care and advised him on nutrition for cartilage growth.

Infant's Injuries Lead to Scoliosis

When an infant is dropped accidentally to the floor on its head or tailbone, the spine can later develop scoliosis. The outcome of early injuries is often not seen until the growing years begin. Mae came to me when she was twelve years old. Her school physical exam had resulted in a diagnosis of scoliosis. My spinal exam and X-ray confirmed scoliosis in her upper and lower back. The standing X-rays of her thoracic and lumbar spine revealed several compression injuries to the vertebral bodies of her mid-thoracic and upper lumbar vertebrae. She had lateral and anterior fractures with a double scoliosis. While reviewing the X-rays, her mother related that she had accidentally dropped Mae several times on her head when she was an infant.

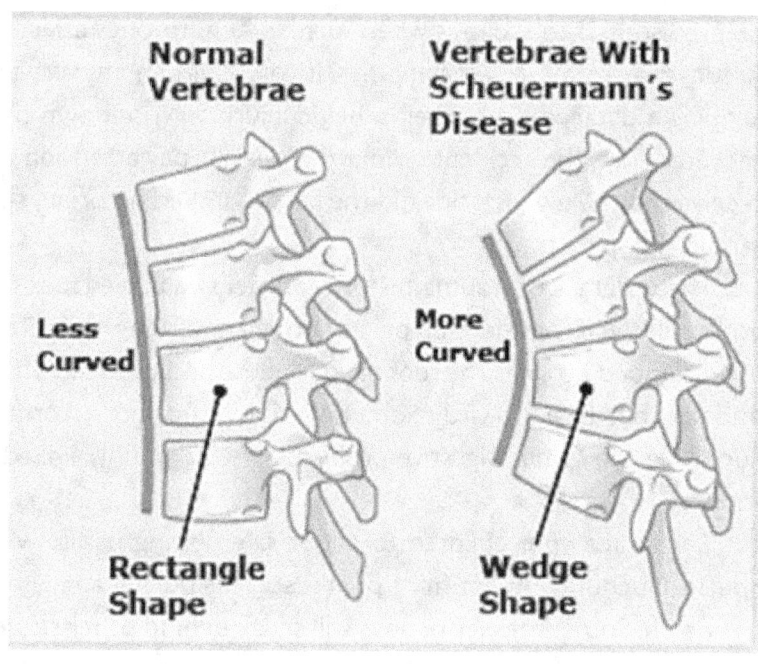

The blood supply to a normal growing vertebral body has end plate symmetry with four branches of arteries feeding the growing plate. Two arteries come across the top sides, right and left, and two more enter the bottom plate on both sides. If a lateral compression trauma damages and constricts blood supply to a portion of the growing plate on one side, the vertebral body will grow in a lopsided fashion. Like a rooftop sloping to the lower wall of a house, the vertebral body does not grow on one side. This takes the normally straight spine and forms the side curvature called scoliosis.

In children the growth plate blood vessels are tiny; even mild trauma can interrupt normal growth patterns. Repetitive falls from skateboards or jumping from heights high enough to crush the end plates of vertebrae often result in poorly developed spines. Cheerleading often leads to side falls, and girls have a greater incidence of scoliosis than boys. Early damage to the side or center of vertebral end plates also damages the intervertebral disc. This leads to irregular cartilage formation and cyst deformities such as cartilage nodes, called Schmorl's nodes.

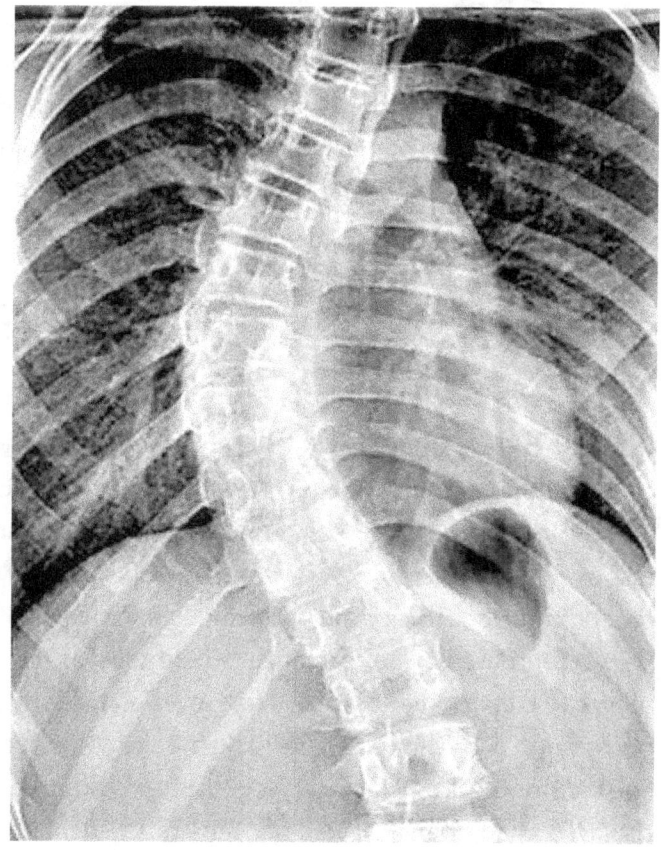

Scoliosis usually develops from physical trauma. While some forms of the condition may have genetic links, most scoliosis derives from injury. Young girls may be predisposed to scoliosis when menstrual hormones affect blood vessel breakdown. Cheerleading and gymnastics may result in spinal injuries. If your children are very active outdoors and in sports, you will benefit by keeping a detailed log of their athletic injuries. Write down the date, the type of activity, how the child's body moved during the accident or injury. Especially pay attention to the position of the spine. Did your child's spine receive a jolt? On which side did the fall occur? Did his or her spine fold over? Which direction, right or left? How far did the spine travel?

These details of trauma history can yield valuable clues that may help formulate beneficial treatments to your children if they develop pain or other conditions years after their sports activities have ended. If your active child climbed up onto the roof of your house and then slid off, record the accident even if injuries are not severe and the child healed swiftly. Sometimes it is difficult to ascertain when a moderate injury has affected the blood supply to the spine. Digestive problems are commonly linked to laterally compressed spines when nerves are irritated.

Encourage your children to adopt safe playing habits whether at home, in parks or in organized school sports. Discourage them from pranks such as pulling a chair out from under a classmate as the other student sits down. Sometimes feisty boys will sneak behind other students and hit the back of their knees, buckling the joint and sending the victim to the ground. Those kids find these antics fun and entertaining, yet abrupt shocks to a child's growing spine can cause interrupted blood supply and consequences such a scoliosis even when no other obvious injury occurs. An injured vertebra may misalign regularly and lead to interrupted functions of the bowel and bladder. A lifelong affliction can result from what appeared to be a harmless practical joke during elementary school.

Parenting skillfully involves guiding your children to make choices along the spectrum of risk when they engage in physical activity. Sports and play that involve high adventure and thrills often come with risk of spinal trauma. Though your child may not have the experience or wisdom to make appropriate choices, she or he may need your support and efforts to steer through childhood with an intact and healthy spine. Certainly, video games and other computer-related activities, while they may entail control of superhero characters that take death defying risks, may not harm a child's spine and lead to scoliosis. But such video play may convince young boys or girls to try similar moves when they jump onto their skateboards, scooters, and bikes, until reality strikes. One injury can lead to a lifetime of illness.

Injury Before Birth

Lisa, a petite young woman in her twenties, came to me when she was performing in a traveling choir. She complained of mid-back pain and restriction. She had suffered from a thoracic scoliosis for several years. We displayed the upper back X-rays she brought in, and I could see how her spine had fatigued. Lisa sought chiropractic care at each city she performed in. She carried her spinal X-rays to each doctor to help relieve her of the pain accentuated by performances where she was required to stand onstage for more than an hour. Lisa came to me for two chiropractic visits. X-rays revealed that she had an underdeveloped or lateral compression fracture to her seventh thoracic vertebrae. I asked if she could recall any trauma that would affect the vertebra at this level. She did not recall any fall or accident that would have injured her spine. I asked her if she had ever fallen or been dropped as an infant. Lisa did not remember such an injury.

Before the second visit she called her mother and asked her about her early life. Her mother had never dropped Lisa, but she told her of a car accident during the last trimester of her pregnancy. Just weeks before giving birth to Lisa, her mother was thrown into the steering wheel during an automobile accident. This may have injured Lisa's backbone before she was even born and formed an unnatural curvature to her spine. It was the first time Lisa had heard this story, and whether it was the cause of the scoliosis, she was grateful to have learned the history. She recounted the story to me on her second visit.

The first signs of spinal trauma that occur at an early age may not appear until the spinal column begins its growth during puberty. Trauma to the spine can occur *in utero*, during the birth process, or pre-puberty to produce an abnormally developing spine. Soft growing bone centers can be separated, twisted, or damaged at birth. Blood supply to growing cartilage and bone can be disrupted. An acute trauma to the spine at the onset of puberty may be severe enough to need surgical intervention if the scoliosis is advancing and the condition unstable. Ninety percent of spinal scoliosis cases do not worsen over time. The shape of the vertebral body can be changed at any time during one's life. However, a lateral compression fracture after the termination of spinal growth not only leads to permanent scoliosis, but a possible onset of serious disease if stem cells bleed out and enter the nerves and tissues.

CHAPTER 6

Intestinal Risks

● ● ●

DRIVER'S SIDE IMPACT LEADS TO COLON CANCER

Six years ago, I met Jeff while attending a seminar on weight loss. An older gentleman about six feet tall with a powerful bone structure much like that of a football player, Jeff was overweight and struggled with his digestive system. Jeff mentioned that years earlier he'd had a section of his colon removed to treat colon cancer. I told Jeff I had been looking for cases of autoimmune disease and cancer since 1985. I was especially interested in injuries that included back pain and vertebral compression fractures leading to stem cell leakage. The most common fractures are found in the thoracic and lumbar spine. Jeff allowed me to take X-rays of his spine in the standing position. Having matched vertebral injury with associated illness 80 percent of the time on X-ray, I was not surprised when I developed the set of films of his lower back. The images revealed a lateral compression fracture on the top left side of his second lumbar vertebra.

Without knowing anything about Jeff's history of injury, I conjectured about how the fracture might have occurred. His spine must have nearly doubled over in some type of accident where his left upper body flexed toward his left hip bone, resulting in compression to the left side of the vertebrae. I suggested as an example that he could have been hit broadside on his driver's side in a car accident. That would account for such an injury. Or he could have fallen hard toward the left side of his body, crunching one vertebra down onto the next. As it turned out, my assumptions based purely on viewing the damages to his spine were uncannily accurate.

Several years earlier Jeff had been sitting in a small car at a red light. When the light turned green, he pulled out into the intersection, and a woman driving a large car plowed into him. The point of impact was his driver's side door. The accident flexed his spine sharply to the left in a range that exceeded normal movement. Jeff's spine was hurt in the accident, and he had no idea what subsequent illnesses would develop over the next several months. Jeff's colon cancer appeared only months after the car accident. A couple of years later he had a portion of the colon removed. He survived, but his health remains tenuous.

After a vertebral compression fracture, stem cells may flow uninterrupted down the sympathetic nerve pathways and enter the base tissue of an organ. Here the stem cells are flowing to the connective tissue of colon.

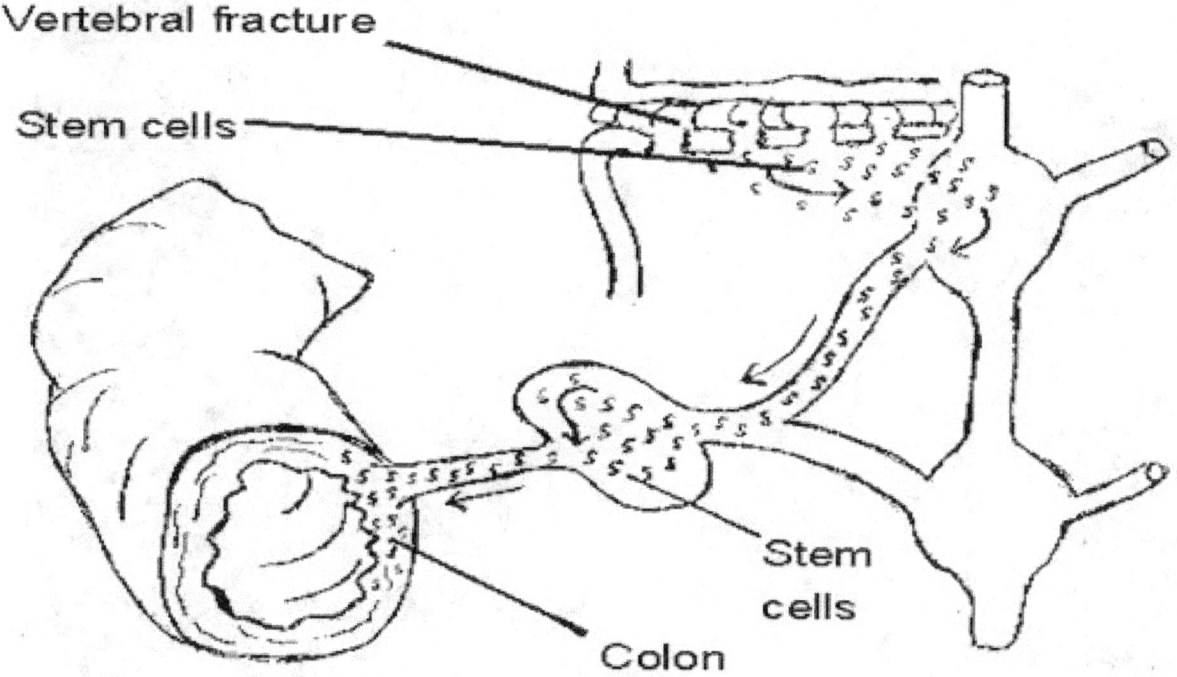

Once the stem cells appear in the connective tissue of the colon, the immune system will react to them as a foreign invader. The resultant inflammation can later evolve into autoimmune disease or the stem cells can change the genetics of the organ's base cells and produce cancer.

Accidents do not have to be severe to damage the spine enough to allow stem cell leakage. All it takes is a tiny crack in the top of the vertebra, especially in an older person whose body cannot wall off or seal the injury to stop leaking stem cells. Stem cells are so small and mobile that they can readily absorb into a nerve where they travel unopposed by the immune system. Jeff may have walked away from this accident shrugging off temporary discomfort, believing that he was lucky, and would not necessarily connect the accident to the subsequent onset of colon cancer.

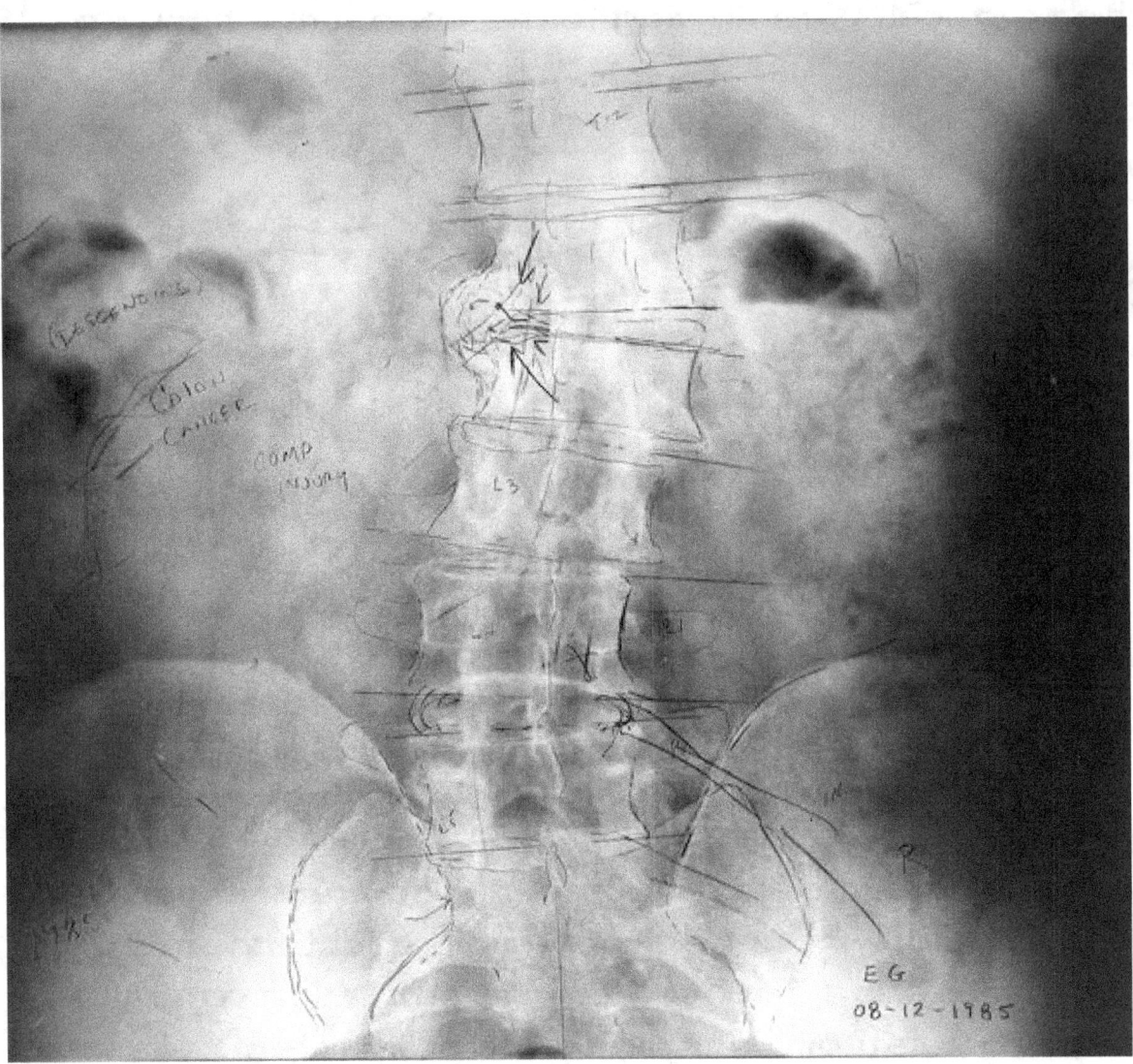

Recent research has revealed that the third process of healing ligament and collagen tissue with calcification may be due in response to stem cells in the region. Could the spine try to contain the stem cell leakage by sealing off the injured area with calcification? In severe injury, the immune system is activated into an immense cascade of healing signals. The immune systems last resort is to wall off, thicken, and mineralize the damaged tissues.

Severe Fall in Supermarket Pushes my Theory

Barry worked as a shift supervisor in a large supermarket in town. After thirty years of employment, one day he walked hurriedly through the produce department. A customer had apparently dropped a few grapes on the floor in the aisle next to the fruit. Even though Barry had passed through that part of the store hundreds of times without incident, that day his shoes skated on the grape skins and his feet flew out from under his body. In a split-second Barry landed hard on his tailbone. The impact fractured the middle of his tailbone – the supporting foundation of the spine. The slip and fall caused his sacrum to fracture into two pieces.

Barry went to an orthopedic physician for treatment. He also came to me in efforts to relieve his lower back pain. After two months of treatment and healing, he returned to work, though within ten months of the sacral fracture he was diagnosed with a rectal colon tumor. Cancer had developed directly in front of the fracture inside of a year's time. Barry had a section of his rectal colon removed and received radiation therapy to arrest further cancer.

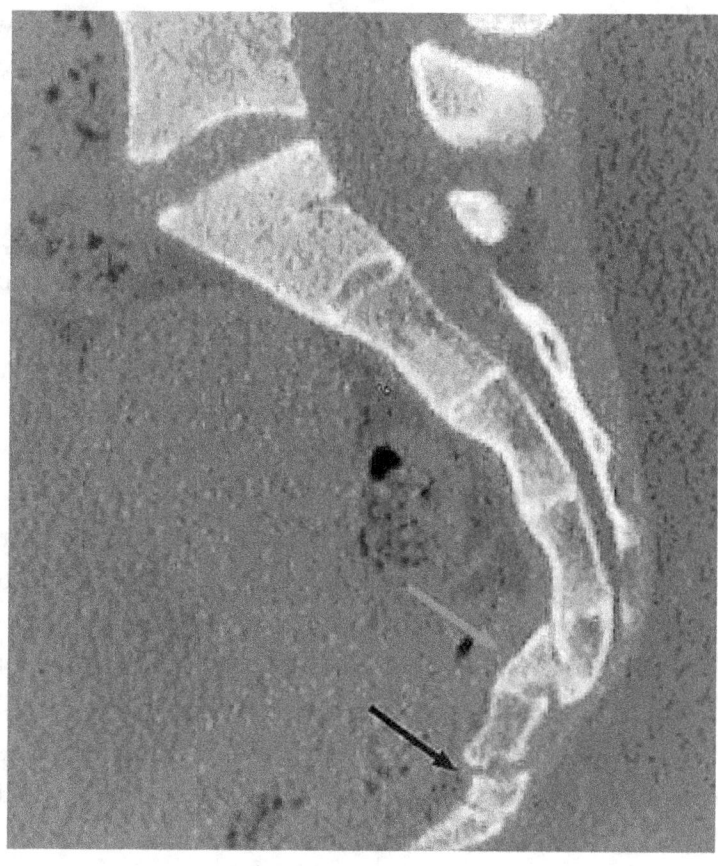

Barry's case – with his specific and localized development of serious disease following spinal trauma – boosted my scientific curiosity to even greater heights. The coincidence of his accident and cancer was difficult to ignore. But what was the link? Through many years of schooling in biochemistry and physiology, I had never seen any discussion of a possible connection between spinal trauma and ailments such as cancer. The rectal tumor was formed directly in front of his sacral fracture. Is it possible that stem cells penetrated the colon tissue after the fracture?

CHILDHOOD ACCIDENT CAUSES COLON DISEASE

If my hypothesis is correct, fractures to the spine that result in leaking stem cells can wreak havoc on the body at any age. The body tries to heal the initial trauma as well as cope with leaked stem cells. Here is a case involving intestinal illness that shows the effects of spinal injury on a young child.

Neil has had ulcerative colitis – bleeding and pain due to autoimmune syndrome in his lower bowels – since he was six years old. The condition caused him considerable embarrassment and many socially awkward moments. Neil's inflamed bowels have bled less in recent years, but the condition plagued him throughout most of his childhood and school years. The malady occurred lower in the colon instead of higher, yet it is still difficult to treat. Treatment through the years has been a cascade of immune suppression medications including prednisone.

Neil's parents had given him a new scooter for his birthday at five years old. Thinking it would be fun, Neil put the bar stem of the scooter behind his back, reaching back to hold the handles. Then he rode the scooter backwards like a skateboard down the sidewalk in his suburban neighborhood. The scooter wheels hit the curb and little Neil went down hard. As he toppled over backwards, the bar of the scooter smashed directly into his tailbone, damaging, or fracturing the back of the tailbone. He had horrible pain. Within a few months he developed a bleeding bowel syndrome known as ulcerative colitis. Stem cells were likely leaked into his intestinal tissue where they did not belong. His immune system attacked the interstitial tissue of the organ, inflaming and destroying the rectal colon collagen support tissue and producing ulcerative colitis.

The phenomenon of collagen breakdown in Neil's colon is not unique to his condition. Heart disease and aneurysms of large arteries are both caused by autoimmune attack. Abnormal widening and thinning of an arterial wall is due to the immune system attacking and removing collagen support tissue. Most autoimmune diseases involve sacrifice of connective tissue or collagen in vital organs. The immune system attacks raw stem cells to render them harmless. Unfortunately, stem cells have genetic resiliency and keep prompting inflammatory responses that develop into chronic illness. Over time, stem cells tend to mutate connective tissue cells into cancer. Then a new war against cancer ensues.

Neil participated in a special study of injection medication for his colitis and bleeding bowels. The goal was to target medication to the affected zone of the body instead of using general medications, which need to go through the liver. The treatment has been partially effective so far. X-rays in 2012 showed that Neil's childhood accident had caused disruption in the mid-sacral segment of the spine. The sacrum is composed of five vertebrae segments that fuse together by the time one is three years old. The sacrum sits below the lowest lumbar vertebra and between the pelvic bones. The tailbone tip or coccyx is located below the sacrum. Because of his damaged sacrum, Neil's illness located itself in the lower part of the colon.

Cases like Neil's are common, though most colon diseases affect older patients. Children and especially adolescent boys sometimes throw themselves into play or sports with such abandon that they put their young bodies at risk in ways an older person would likely avoid. Imagine adolescent children on skateboards or dirt bikes, making daredevil spins and somersaults, riding over steps, and leaping concrete walls. These activities promote an adventurous spirit that may promote a mistaken sense of immortality. Inevitable crashes from their stunts can sadly lead to lifetime afflictions with their intestinal tracts.

One compression fracture in a lumbar vertebra from a skateboard disaster can ruin the rest of a young child's life. One hard tumble from a girl galloping on her horse through rough rocky terrain can spoil her digestion for decades or prompt reproductive disorders that interfere with childbearing potential. Especially with adults, I have linked over 300 cases of vertebral compression injury that occurred before the onset of intestinal illness.

Growth hormone, present in children during puberty, often allows them to miraculously heal spinal trauma, but does not resolve the irritable bowel syndrome or other maladies that develop in their intestines. In people under twenty years of age, growth hormone allows them to better seal off areas of leaking stem cells, limiting subsequent destructive effects. Once patients have finished puberty, the story changes dramatically as healing factors are less available.

Internal organs have no pain alert mechanisms to signal to a person that something has gone terribly wrong in the gut. Colon cancer may progress quite far without any symptoms at all. The intervertebral disc has a large amount of pain sensation in its posterior walls. However, the fractured bone has no pain sensation on the inside of its structure. Spinal sensation is crucial to overall body functioning. Our bodies are designed to signal a high alert with even a mild disc injury. However, a small vertebral fracture may produce little to no pain yet be the beginning of a serious illness.

Heavy Construction Work and Bladder Cancer

George came into my office at age forty-five. He had chronic lower back pain and deteriorating lumbar discs from working heavy construction since he was a teen. He had worked hard as a road paver and operated big equipment. His body was broken down from lifting thousands of pounds of construction supplies, and from endless hours of sitting and twisting in the seats of tractors and earthmovers. His spine withstood years of stooping, bending, pushing, and pulling. While performing his physical exam, George told me he recently had been diagnosed with bladder cancer. X-rays were taken that day not only for the position of his vertebrae and disc stability, but also for examining his bone integrity.

The standing lumbar x-rays revealed a lateral disc protrusion to the left side of segments lumbar 1 to lumbar 2. It included a lateral compression fracture to the top left side of his lumbar 2 vertebra. When I reviewed the X-rays with George, he told me how years earlier he had fallen over to the right while operating a backhoe. His spine bent over to the side with the weight of the equipment nearly crushing him. His lower back has never been the same since. Injuries to the left side of the first three lumbar vertebrae have coincided in my studies usually with colon cancer, colon disease, prostate cancer, bladder cancer and female reproductive cancer and disease.

What was revealed on George's X-rays, along with recent research on inflammatory proteins causing neuritis and pain, made me contemplate the molecular size of protein. The 1980s research brought inflammatory proteins under closer scrutiny. Collagen protein of joint and disc cartilage, when broken down, was found to be absorbed into pain receptors, which then signal pain to our brains. These proteins not only signaled pain as cells were damaged, but they also passed easily into connective tissues, triggering the immune system into operation. Small proteins were able to absorb into nerve endings for pain sensation; why couldn't they pass into nerves and travel downstream to the organ tissues? Studies were proving that leg pain was due more to absorption of small inflammatory proteins than to compressed nerves. Nerve inflammation, called neuritis, can inflame an entire leg, or individual regions.

If a drop of poison can take a life, how could something so small cause such a huge range of cell death? As proteins are broken down, they return to their smallest parts. Proteins are built from small genetic molecules. New research was showing that nerves not only had electrical impulses, they also had tiny proteins flowing down the center inside microtubules along the axon. Then it came to me. Stem cells are so small, if raw and undifferentiated, they must be able to absorb through a damaged nerve lining and migrate along its pathway. Tiny stem cells, once inside the center of a nerve, can travel untouched by the immune system and flow into the framework of organs. Stem cells are attacked and recycled at the injury site by local immune cells, blood, and lymph channels. If my idea is correct, red bone marrow stem cells that enter and flow down a nerve axon end up directly in the organ support tissue — which is the battleground of all autoimmune diseases and the production sites for cancer.

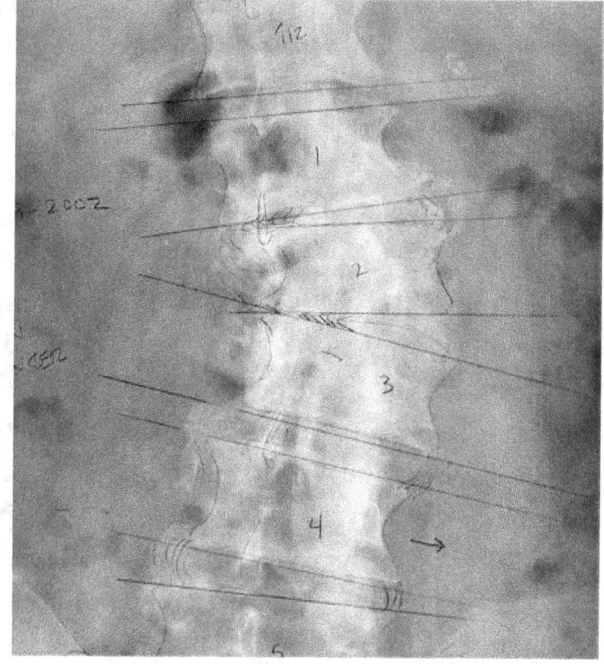

In my personal research cases, over eighty percent of the time a vertebral compression fracture coincided with a post-traumatic serious illness. The spinal fractures were **never** due to cancer of the vertebra. Despite what other researchers might think, these cases were not due to metastasis to the spine. In a few cases where the patient's doctor determined that cancer had spread to a vertebra, a previous compression injury had occurred. Just by viewing hundreds of x-rays and MRI images of spinal cancer on the internet, I can see one main compression fractured vertebrae. The other vertebrae with metastasis appear above or below the fracture. These cases were due to a specific trauma at a specific time. Where most cancers developed over weeks or months, some cases of cancer and autoimmune disease I dealt with were diagnosed within days of the injury.

As my ideas have evolved, I am now sharing stories in what are over 700 cases with doctors and professionals. I knew there would be a time where I could pull this information together as a coherent theory of the genesis of certain types of disease. I still choose not to write medical reviewed articles. I just keep pushing for more cases. Stem cells cause illness, I have no doubt. My theory that stem cells serve as the catalyst to disease was boosted by considerable research in the 1990s. Research news articles warned the public of the detrimental effects of using stem cells for treatment. Try an Internet search for any disease and add the words "stem cell" in the query. Search far past all the stem cell therapy promises and you will see that stem cells have been implicated at the center of many diseases. The following case contains other parallel events along with vertebral fractures that lead to illness.

FOOTBALL INJURY LEADS TO CROHN'S DISEASE

Bart was a standout for the Stanford University football team. A lanky man who stood nearly 6'5" in height, Bart was an experienced wide receiver. Driven with ambition, he played hard. During one play at the apex of his football career, Bart went out for a crucial pass in a game with the score tied late in the fourth quarter. He leaped high into the air and caught the football, but at that moment a defensive player nailed him hard with a flying tackle. Bart crashed to the turf when the other football player's body pounded into his torso. The impact violently folded his spine and collapsed him sideways. The punishing tackle caused a lateral compression fracture to the right side of his thoracic vertebra. He recovered and continued to play, possibly resulting in further injury to the mid-back vertebrae. Within a few months after the fracture injury, Bart developed colitis and Crohn's disease in his small intestine. The condition plagued him for the rest of his life.

For more than forty years after his college football career ended, Bart fought irritable bowel syndrome and Crohn's disease into his late sixties. He became a patient of mine in his early fifties. Bart had a long thoracic spine with steeply angled scoliosis, or lateral curvature. The football injury most likely led to a lateral compression fracture and his subsequent autoimmune disease. X-rays revealed that the compression fracture was in the region where I have seen dozens of colitis cases. But this case doesn't just end in an autoimmune disease of the intestines. The condition moved on to cancer like so many other colitis conditions I have seen.

Bart received relief for his back pain and colitis with my chiropractic treatments over several years. I examined his spine monthly. Then one day during an office visit Bart pointed to a one-inch square growth off the side of his ribs. I told him to have it examined immediately. I thought is to be serious, as it was at the same vertebral level as his old thoracic spinal fracture. I had seen skin lesions above the site of vertebral fractures many times. He received a biopsy and was diagnosed with squamous cell skin cancer. The cancer had already spread to the rest of his body.

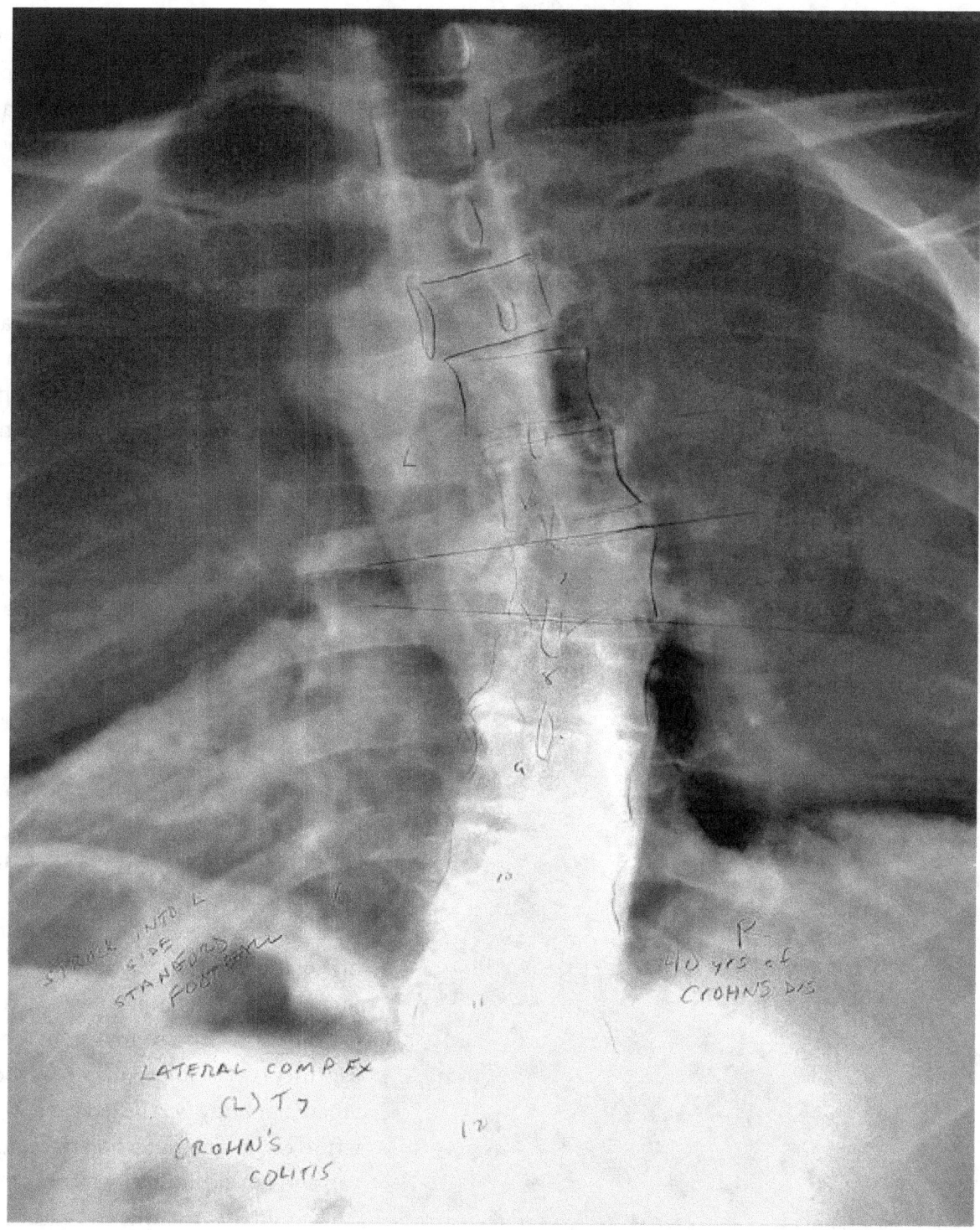

The image above reveals the football clipping vertebral trauma that led to a player's Crohn's disease. Interesting, I have found a lateral compression fracture in almost every Crohn's case I ever examined. Some end plate compression changes are not as obvious as this one.

Bart received an experimental chemotherapy drug that unfortunately caused an infection in his brain and produced a coma. He emerged from the coma, but the cancer took his life within a few months. Is it possible that the cancer developed as a late response to the earlier bleeding of stem cells? Could the chronic autoimmune attack of the small intestine have mutated his colon tissue into a cancerous stage, such as squamous cell cancer?

RANCHING INJURY CAUSES ENDOMETRIOSIS

Renee, a twenty-year-old college student, arrived at my office complaining of left lower back spasm, pain, and restriction from her left upper lumbar vertebrae down to the sacrum. At Renee's initial examination and treatment, her mother was in attendance. No X-rays were taken at the time of the first visit. During the examination at her second visit, her mother explained that her daughter had menstrual "bleeding all the time." It had been a problem for five years. I told her she might have a lateral lumbar fracture which can lead to a condition called endometriosis, an autoimmune disease of the uterus. With her permission I took standing lumbar x-rays during the second visit, searching for a compression injury to the left side of the first two upper lumbar vertebrae. The x-rays revealed a mild left lateral compression fracture of the second lumbar vertebrae. At her third visit to my office, viewed the X-ray findings. I pointed out the lateral compression fracture and explained to them my stem cell leakage theory. An injury may have occurred where her body was flexed violently to the left to cause a compression fracture on the top and left side of the vertebra.

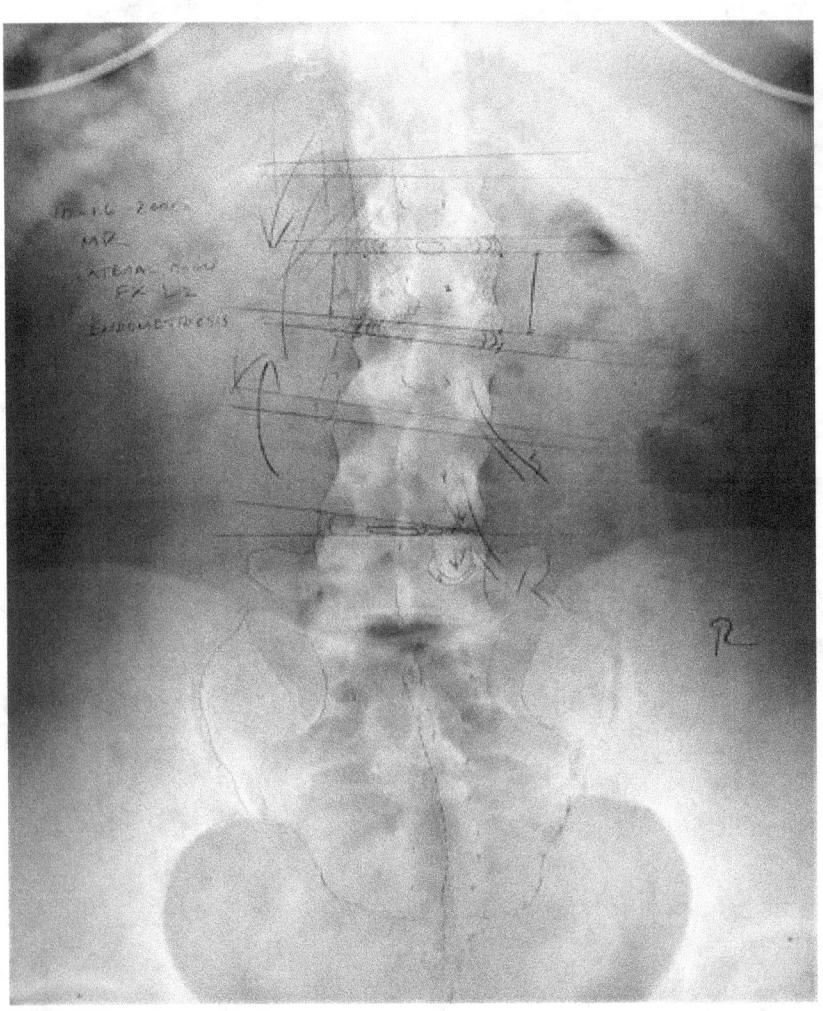

During the treatment, I gave examples how this injury might have happened. Renee suddenly stopped me, exclaiming she knew how it occurred. She recalled having worked with a heifer that weighed several hundred pounds. The heifer slipped and fell, pushing and bending Renee to the left side as the cow fell on top of her. This could easily have been the cause of the compression fracture. It had happened five years prior and matched up with the beginning of her bleeding menses condition. Subsequent examinations and treatments helped her lower back condition but were only mildly useful for her symptoms of endometriosis.

Of over 700 of patient cases who have suffered compression fracture to the spine, almost a third developed some malady of the small or large intestine, which includes the colon. Some of these cases developed into colon cancer, while others settled into a chronic irritated colon that caused significant and life-ruining discomfort. Maladies such as Crohn's disease damage the small intestine and interfere with digestion. Cancer of the small intestine is not as common.

Colorectal cancer risks can arise from a variety of contributing factors in addition to the possible link to bleeding stem cells from nearby spinal injury. Nearly one in four people over age fifty have weak colon walls and polyps. Nearly 150,000 new cases of colorectal cancer are diagnosed in the United States each year. Consumption of alcohol and cigarette smoking may increase colon disease, along with obesity and lack of exercise. Dietary factors such as animal fat and fiber, especially for those with diabetes, also play a role. As with many illnesses, genetics and family background may affect our digestive health.

Among my patients with Crohn's disease and colon cancer, about 80 percent have had lateral compression fractures or lateral disc protrusions within the thoracic or lumbar spine. Fractures over the right side of the thoracic vertebrae lead to inflammation of the small intestine or Crohn's disease. Fractures of the upper lumbar vertebrae or sacrum lead to ulcerative colitis or cancer of the colon. Numerous sympathetic nerves find their way to the connective tissues of the intestines. These nerves are the possible roadways for leaked stem cells to migrate and enter the intestinal tissues.

SAME SPINAL INJURY LEVELS PRODUCE THE SAME DISEASE

Mike, an active ocean diver and bowler, like myself, came to me at age forty-three. He suffered from irritable bowel syndrome and had had a foot-long section of his intestine removed about two years earlier. Mike fractured two of his lower thoracic vertebrae two years prior to his surgery in an accident related to hunting. He was driving an all-terrain vehicle in the hills when he lost control of the vehicle. It flipped over, falling on top of him and folding him under. This the accident led to the vertebral compression fracture of his thoracic vertebrae.

Patricia, a high school biology teacher, arrived at my office with chronic lower back pain and a history of colitis. She was a patient in her fifties and told me of a severe injury of falling down stairs when she was in her thirties. I located the injury by taking lumbar spinal X-rays. Patricia had a lateral compression injury with a laterally herniated disc to the

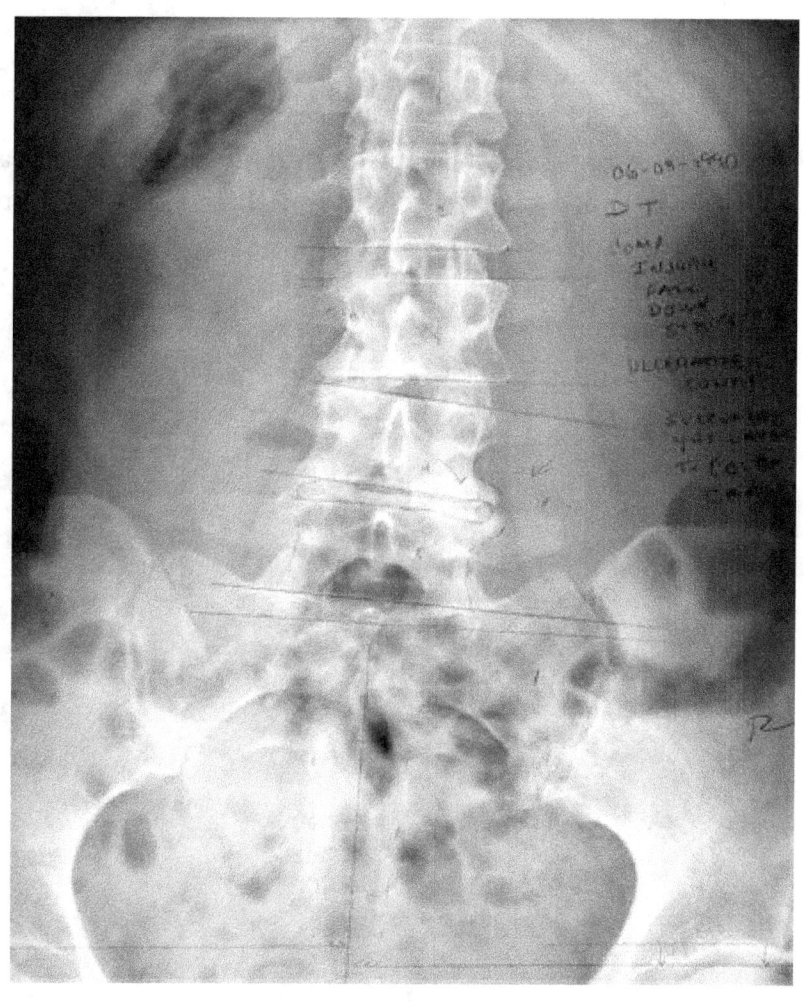

sides of the lumbar vertebrae. She had had lower back pain and restriction of back movement for years after the accident. Patricia said she suffered colitis ever since the fall type injury. The lateral disc protrusion and compression injury may have produced autoimmune disease in her colon. Patricia had scoliosis, a lateral curve of the spine. I found out a year after I had treated her that she had subsequently progressed into colon cancer. Patricia succumbed to colon cancer before the age of sixty.

Sometimes dermatological signs signal deeper troubles in the body relating to spinal trauma from decades earlier. Marilyn, a dairy owner in her eighties, received treatment every month for chronic lower back pain. She had multiple compressed discs in her lumbar spine as evident on my spinal x-rays. Over several years of observation and treatment, I watched a two-inch square light browned skin pigmentation change to a darker color on her lower back. I had her notify her doctors of the condition. The skin lesion was near the left side of her upper two lumbar vertebrae. As the patch of skin began turning darker, Marilyn began having more bowel problems. It looked like early signs of melanoma. Eventually Marilyn was diagnosed with colon cancer, which took her life. The change in skin pigmentation was located where the spine had trauma. It served as a warning of impending cancer. Melanoma, once it appears on the skin, may have already resulted in metastasis to other vital organs such as the lungs, brain, or liver, and often leads to death. I observed this same skin change in a couple other patients who had compression trauma to their spines.

A person, who has avoided the misfortune of having spinal injury and fracture often enjoys a much better quality of life throughout later years. Another patient named Joe recently reached 100 years of age. He has come to my office for twenty-two years for minor backaches and pains. His X-rays reveal little arthritis and no compression fractures. He has no deteriorative arthritis. A hard-working dairy rancher, Joe milked cows until he was eighty-six years old. His memory and cognitive functions are extraordinarily sharp as a centenarian.

Most of my patients who live comfortably into their eighties and nineties have no significant spinal injuries. They were lucky to avoid damage to the vertebrae and subsequent deterioration of organ function. Some people have developed disease or cancer relatively quickly after a vertebral compression fracture. Anterior compression fractures and arch fractures of the vertebrae can also leak out stem cells. Stem cells can bleed into the tissues behind the heart or lungs, or into the organs of the abdominal cavity. This can lead to systemic lupus or a catastrophic immune response of complete organ systems.

CHAPTER 7

Heart and Lung Disease

• • •

AUTOIMMUNE DISEASE OCCURS AT THE interstitial level of cell structure - the base tissue that composes the organ. Collagen fibers of sulfur-based proteins make up the framework of organs. When autoimmune disease occurs, it happens almost exclusively within this tissue, and typically starts to destroy the connective collagen. Why? Autoimmune disease may start from a lateral vertebral fracture located next to the beginning branch of the sympathetic nerve. After such a fracture, leaked stem cells may enter the autonomic nerves of the sympathetic nervous system. The distal pathways of these nerves lead to the interstitial tissues of organs.

In the various types and locations of autoimmune disease, the tissue consumed by and ultimately destroyed by our own immune cells is the structural connective tissues — not the specialized cells that make up the organ. If immune cells attacked the specialized cell tissue, there would be quick loss of organ function. Instead, loss of form occurs slowly, often through dilation as our white blood cells devour our own connective tissues and the organ expands. Aneurysms, bowel dilatation, leaking gut and loss of structure of the kidney and heart are due to our own immune cells thinning and consuming our sulfur-based tissue.

Why does the initial attack involve fibers of collagen? Could this be the location, the entrance points of leaked stem cells? Are the leaked stem cells so undeveloped that the immune system identifies them as small viruses? Stem cells, raw and untouched as they flow through autonomic nerves may be reacted to by the immune system as foreign invaders. The body, alarmed at the invasion, produces inflammation. Stem cells are so small, like viruses, that they produce an antigenic and allergic reaction against your own body's cells. This reaction can happen if you consume your own species' connective tissues. Cows were fed ground up organ tissue of their own species, an autoimmune complex occurred called mad cows disease. The same immune system disorder was reproduced by a researcher at UCSF in San Francisco, California when he fed chickens the ground up organs of their own species. The mechanism of autoimmune disease is very complex and not yet fully understood.

BALES OF HAY COMPRESS MIDDLE BACK

The entrance of large numbers of stem cells into the tissues can happen following an anterior compression fracture of the vertebral body. Compression fractures that occur because of deep spinal flexion can release stem cells and other marrow components into the body cavity and organs located in front of those vertebrae. In recent terms the subsequent immune reaction is now known as a Catastrophic Immune Response. It is likely due to a large quantity of stem cells bleeding into the thoracic or abdomen cavity, overwhelming the immune system.

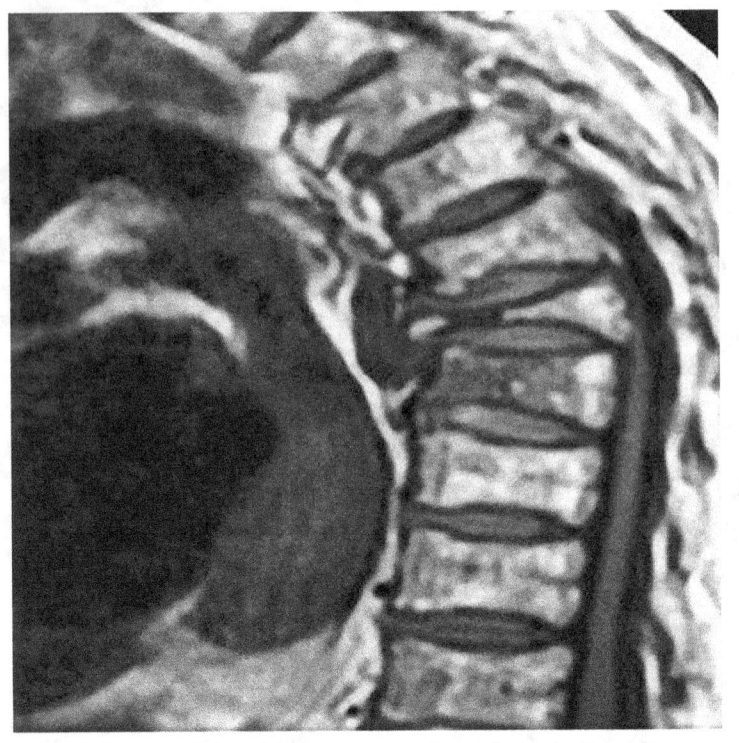

Take the case of Allen, a longtime farmer of alfalfa hay production. In his early sixties, after turning over his family business to his sons, he was involved in a serious accident on the ranch. A bale of hay stacked fifteen feet high slid off and fell onto Allen's back, pressing his spine toward the ground. The weight of the bale tumbling down crushed his spine together. The hyper-flexion injury caused a forward compression fracture of his mid-thoracic vertebrae. The two vertebrae involved were directly located behind his heart and lungs. By the fourth day, Allen was diagnosed with autoimmune attack of his heart and lungs. Doctors told him to save his life, he would need a heart and lung transplant, or he may succumb to a catastrophic immune response within a couple of days. The heart and lung disease happened fast: his immune cells over-reacted to the bleeding injury and produced an autoimmune response within hours of the trauma. Doctors and specialists applied immune suppressant therapy to prolong his life, and within two years Allen had succumbed from his injury.

RIB FRACTURES AND SARCOMA TUMOR OF THE HEART

Another patient, Doris, was under my treatment for years. I had known Doris as a young woman; her family was on my egg route. She suffered from common lower-back and mid-back pain. On an X-ray of her thoracic spine, there was an old fracture injury at the end of a rib where it joins with the vertebra. This injury occurred just behind the heart, and happened when she fell onto her back, landed on a large rock, and fractured the rib. The accident happened in her late teens. The rib injury caused chronic pain for her along with lower back pain. The vertebral segments next to the damaged rib never had proper motion after she had the trauma.

After years of successful treatment to give these thoracic vertebrae motion and better position, Doris came into my office with alarming news. She had been very ill for days, and her doctors were studying her heart. They concluded that she had a sarcoma tumor of her heart located right where her past trauma to the rib and vertebrae had occurred. Could it be that a battle had taken place over several years where stem cells that entered the framework of her heart invoked a genetic change in heart tissue, which finally showed up as cancer?

SECOND BACK FUSION SURGERY AND SARCOMA CANCER

Cancer of muscle tissue is rare, but here is another case. Kay lived in town, but she loved horses and open country. She rode her horse Minney after school and on weekends. Not interested in riding competition or show, Kay galloped through hill and valleys into remote areas most city folk had never seen. One bright spring morning, Kay was riding Minney at full gallop, enjoying the athleticism of the horse. Minney suddenly stopped. Kay could not hold on and was thrown to the ground on her right hip. Her body folded as she rolled over a few times. Kay was in excruciating pain that day and for weeks that followed. X-rays of her lower spine revealed a lateral compression fracture and transverse process fracture of the fourth lumbar vertebra.

Kay was never the same after that injury in her late teens. She stopped riding. Sitting or standing at work was uncomfortable, and the pain became chronic. Lower back and leg pain had fully disrupted her life. Kay came to my office in her mid-twenties. The spinal care I administered was partially effective. Treatment with chiropractic and physical therapy kept Kay on the job until her early thirties. She had another injury to the same region of her lower back caused by lifting heavy items. With conservative treatment becoming less effective, her orthopedic doctors recommended back surgery.

The back surgery recommended to Kay was a full discectomy of the discs between lumbar four and lumbar five, and also between lumbar five and the sacrum. The procedure required fusion of the two vertebrae together and to the sacrum. Bone fragments scraped from her pelvic bone would be used to create the fusion.

Kay went through the surgery and was slow to heal. Months later the leg and back pain were still not alleviated. On further examination, her orthopedic surgeons declared the first surgery a failure and recommended that the fusion surgery be redone. The leg pain had become horrible again, and Kay was losing more time at work. She agreed to redo the fusion surgery but was not prepared for what would happen next. Following the second back surgery, Kay developed sarcoma cancer along the left side of her paraspinal and erectors spinalis muscle groups. The cancer extended from the point of surgery all the way up to just below her left shoulder blade. It was a horrible disfiguring cancer that destroyed her back muscle and overlaying skin. When Kay returned to my office after the second failed back surgery, she had scar tissue the full length of the left side of her back.

I pondered the process of her surgery. With the back muscles cut open and pulled back during the operation, could it be that as the surgeon cut the arch of the lumbar vertebrae for a second time, stem cells bled into the muscle tissue? Or when the surgeon brought the bone material into place, stem cells were inadvertently absorbed into the muscle tissue? Recent research has proven that bone grafting materials from the patient or a donor can lead to cancer in and around the surgical graft.

The resulting sarcoma tumor was so specific and so far up the multifidus muscle that stem cells entering the fascia and muscle of the back may have set off an immune attack which evolved into cancer. The difference between remaining as an active autoimmune inflammation and converting into cancer occurs when the stem cell makes a genetic change. If the attack of the immune system is insufficient over time, stem cells may overtake the connective tissue cells, mutating or making a genetic flip to enhance the stem cells' survival. Once the flip occurs and cancer begins, the immune system must deal with a hungry set of dividing cancer cells. The immune system plays a part in destroying tissue too, ahead of the cancer's direction of growth. Large amounts of tissues may be destroyed, losing structure and then function. Although cancer mostly involves the support or connective tissues of organs, at times the specialized cells or muscle cells are also involved, as in sarcoma. The result for Kay was another failed back surgery, and a major loss of muscle mass that ended up as thick uneven scar tissue.

Professional Ice Skater Falls and Fractures Back

At a recent chiropractic conference, I was discussing my theory with a few chiropractors who graduated around the same time. One doctor sought to learn more about my ideas. After hearing my idea that stem cells cause autoimmune disease and cancer, she told me about a case which matched my theory. She and her husband are both chiropractors in a large city where there is a major ice rink used for hockey and ice skating. One of her patients, a professional ice skater, had a serious fall on the ice.

The patient had compression fractures of the twelfth thoracic and first lumbar vertebrae. Immediately after this trauma, the female patient went into autoimmune disease and inflammation of her kidneys, pancreas, and liver. The skater most likely had substantial leakage of stem cells into the upper abdomen quadrant and sympathetic nerves supplying these organs. The doctor was amazed and agreed with my conclusion.

Recently a chiropractor classmate of mine read my first book Stem Cells and Spinal Trauma. He agreed with the association of illness after trauma to the spine and had a more personal case to discuss. He sat me down and told me that his thirty-eight-year-old daughter had been suffering bowel and abdominal illnesses for twenty years. At age eighteen she was thrown and fell from her horse. She had fractured the first lumbar vertebra in the fall. The doctor subsequently updated me that his daughter is now diagnosed with systemic lupus. Even as I write this revised edition, I have received several more cases of lupus and autoimmune diseases such as ulcerative colitis directly related to falls from a horse and traumatic lifting injury.

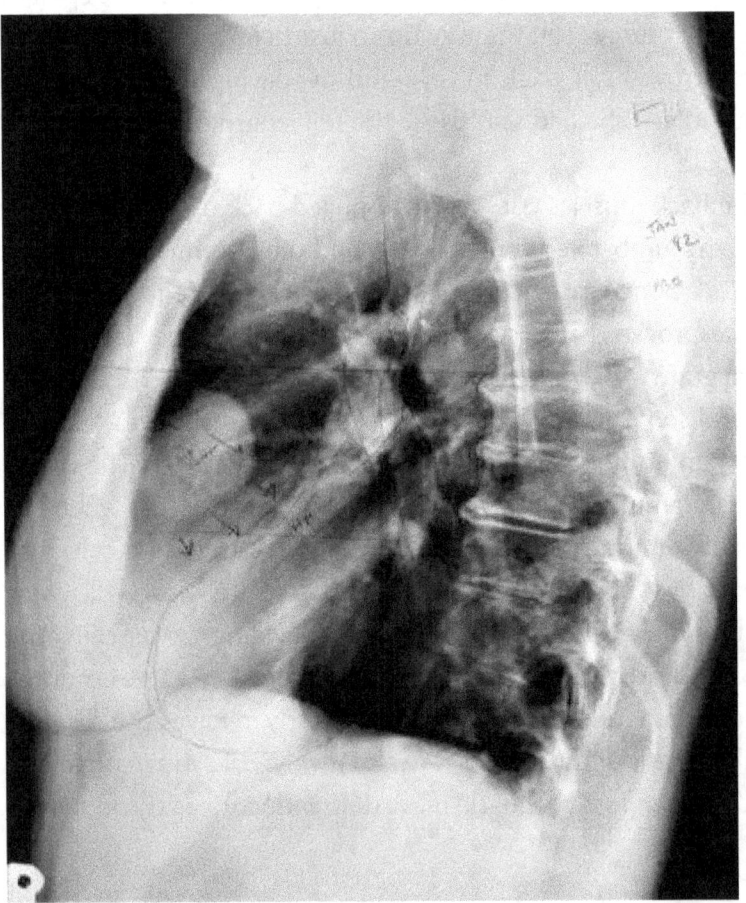

Past Compression Injury and Heart Disease

One winter when Laila was in her late teens, she suffered a compression injury to her mid-thoracic vertebrae while riding a sled downhill in winter snow. She hurtled into a ditch and her mid-back was compressed downward. In her early fifties she began examinations for what turned out to be heart disease. On an X-ray examination, doctors found that Laila had a tumor under her sternum that was compressing the front of her heart. Before the growth was removed, I took thoracic X-rays. On the lateral view the tumor was easily visible. What interested me was how the three compressed vertebrae with their irregularly shaped vertebral plates almost exactly delineated the tumor in front. The top injured vertebrae and the bottom injured vertebrae aligned with the top and bottom of the tumor. Could this be a latent effect of stem cell leakage? Were Laila's heart disease and tumor caused by an early injury that led to a failed system? Don't forget the story I told about the catastrophic immune response with the rancher who had compression fractures behind his heart, due to bales of hay striking his upper back.

CAN RIB FRACTURES LEAD TO BREAST AND LUNG CANCER?

An injury that produces fractured ribs can be a simple crack or a complete and separated fracture. Separated or open bleeding rib fractures have a higher chance of bleeding out stem cells. Rib fractures are painful and can be surgically mended if severe, but most heal within one or two months. Not only do stem cells from vertebral fractures enter tissues and cause cancer, I believe, rib fractures could do the same to surrounding lymph nodes and lung tissues. Do fractured ribs bleed out stem cells into blood rich lung tissue? If so, does a minute fracture leak enough stem cells to produce lung illness? Does it take a complete fracture of the rib to bleed out sufficient stem cells to produce illness? Since 1985, I have related dozens of cases of rib fractures with associated serious illness.

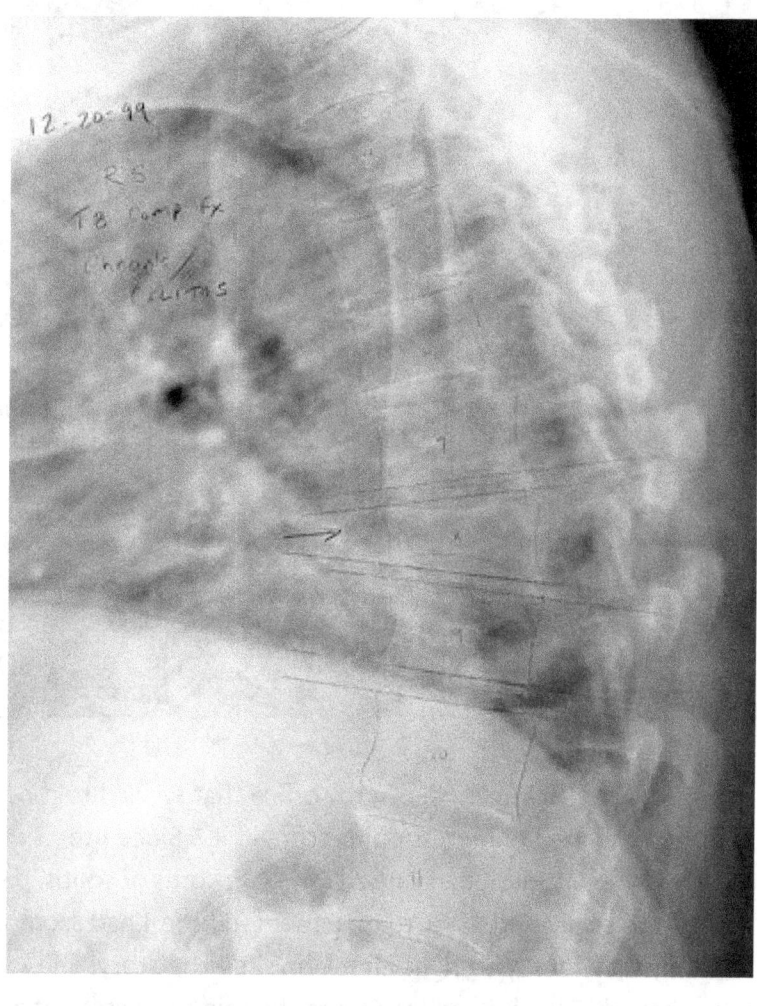

I have associated several cases of rib fractures with lymphoma. The patients had no previous diagnosis of cancer, and there was no cancer adjacent to the rib to have been the cause of the fracture. Stem cells are linked to lymphoma. However, lymphocytes have many possible environmental and lifestyle enemies that can mutate its base codes into cancer. Since cancer of the lung can evade early diagnosis, there can be a pre-pathology that weakened the rib's bone structure. Yet I have seen cases where healthy middle-aged people have fallen, fractured their ribs and ended up with lymphoma cancer within two months of their injury. Sternal fractures can also bleed out stem cells as it contains red bone marrow.

Compression type fractures and other injuries to thoracic vertebrae may lead to conditions such as autoimmune disease of the bronchial, liver, pancreas, small intestines, and lung tissues. Depending on the immune system's failure or success, the stem cell disease may progress into cancer and damage the liver, stomach, lung, and pancreas. The degree of damage depends on the person's healing ability. For some patients, injuries that initiated autoimmune disease in the small intestines such as Crohn's disease later evolved into intestinal cancer. Right sided upper thoracic injuries result in bronchial problems, or if the injury releases a greater number of stem cells, asthma can develop.

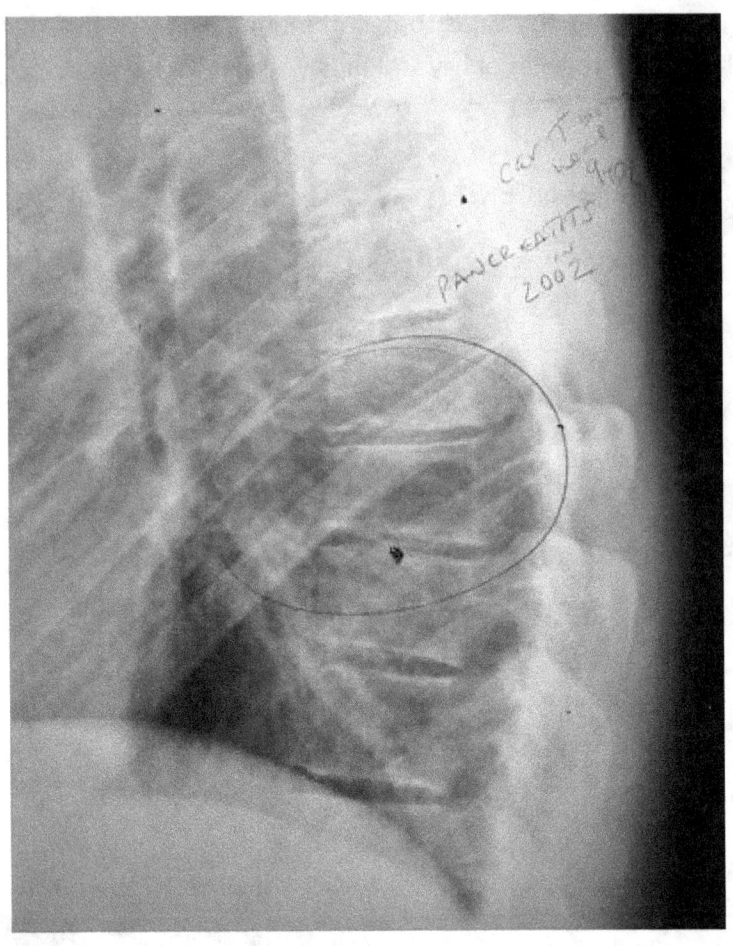One of the most common association of spinal fracture and disease involves a right lateral compression fracture at the vertebral body of T7. One patient in his mid-twenties had a compression fracture to thoracic vertebra seven and developed acute pancreatitis for six months. Another person in his late forties fell from a ladder and compressed the same vertebra then died in thirty days from pancreatic cancer. The first young man had an alcohol problem, the second man had a drug addiction. Yet a third case of many, deals with a nurse practitioner originally worked for my medical physician. She had taken a new position in Kaiser and worked in the ER. Dealing with my mother's final days of life, I had to have her sent by ambulance to the Kaiser Hospital's ER. To my surprise, I'll call her Kelly, was my mom's ER nurse for the first day. As she cared for my mom, she took my mind away by asking what I was up to. I told her about my book and my theory regarding stem cells causing cancer. One time when she stepped back into the room, I gave her three patient case examples of my idea. The last case I spoke of involved a man in his late twenties who just came back in my office that week. I told her I placed his thoracic x-rays on the view box and reviewed the mild compression fracture at T7. Since I took the x-rays five years earlier, I wondered again if the truck rollover accident had caused any symptoms of colitis, pancreatitis, or Crohn's disease. He spoke up immediately and exclaimed, "Don't you remember doc, I had six months of pancreatitis after the rollover accident!"

Kelly's jaw dropped right after I finished the story! She said, "I believe in your theory!" I was surprised and asked her why? With a saddened face she told me a story of a couple she knows that she just ran into last week. Kelly said the husband was pale, thin, and looked emaciated. She asked what was up. The wife told her that two months prior they were on a trip in Australia and wound up in serious automobile accident. She told Kelly her husband fractured T7, thoracic 7, and subsequently developed pancreatic cancer. I was so sorry to hear this, informed Kelly on some nutritional advice and never forgot how she felt about my findings. The x-ray above reveals another automobile accident with pancreatitis. The sympathetic supply to the pancreas is most likely greater at the right side of T7.

CHAPTER 8

Melanoma and Brain Tumors

• • •

THE BASE LAYER OF OUR skin is 75 percent collagen, which holds vessels and all skin cells in place. Near the base of skin, mixed with skin collagen, are melanocytes. Melanocytes produce pigmenting substances of our skin. They release pigment proteins into the matrix of collagen fibers to help attract sunlight for Vitamin D production and protect us from sun damage. The pigments are known as melanin; collagen cells are known as keratinocytes. Melanocytes form differing pigments that make up the varieties of skin colors.

Melanin protects the skin by absorbing harmful UVA and UVB rays in sunlight. Melanin deposited into the protein of hair produces the varieties of hair color. When production of melanin pigment is stopped or insufficient, skin becomes pale and without color. When production of melanin pigment is in excess, skin is darkened and can turn black. Studies related to the effects of sunlight in damaging our skin are well-known. DNA or genetic damage may occur with certain wavelengths of sunlight. The next couple of stories may lead to more investigation into tagging stem cells as antigens and mutagens when they escape undeveloped following spinal trauma.

SWIMMING ACCIDENT PRODUCES MELANOMA AND BRAIN TUMORS

Sally, one of my patients over years earlier was a high school physical education teacher and swim coach. I found out from other patients that Sally was in serious ill health with melanoma cancer and brain tumors. I thought of her daily and found myself running into her husband down town. He was also a patient and he knew of my ideas of spinal injury and cancer. After he filled me in on Sally's poor health condition, I asked him if she had any recent injury or spinal fracture. I was amazed at how his facial expression changed as he told me she had just injured her back two months prior while swimming. Sally had performed a flip turn too close to the wall and struck the back of her neck and upper back into the wall of the pool. She noticed a skin lesion appeared weeks later on her upper back where she struck the spine. The melanoma pigmentation appeared just above the vertebra she had fractured. I told her husband to bring her in for an evaluation and x-rays.

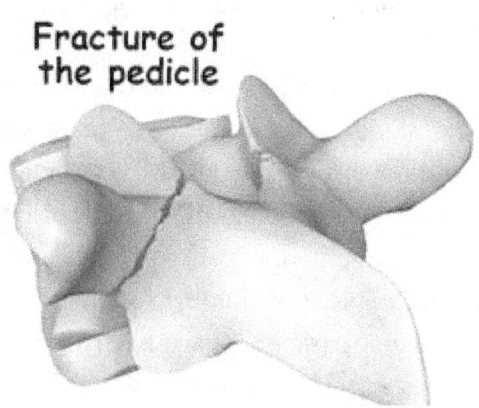
Fracture of the pedicle

X-rays images can evaluate what are called vertebral arch or pedicle fractures. These fractures are fairly easy to see on the neck on obliques views. The CT scans can help diagnosis these fractures, especially in the thoracic and lumbar spine. Besides the possible flow of stem cells from a posterior arch fracture into the dermal nerve branches, in Sally case the stem cell bleeding may have entered the spinal cords fluids and ascended to the brain. She had developed brain tumors weeks the injury along with the melanoma. I cared for and treated Sally for pain until the end of her life.

Escaped adult stem cells from the marrow in a fractured vertebral arch, joint pillar or vertebral body can flow into nerves leading to the skin. If the immune system cannot handle incoming stem cells, the autoimmune reaction may lead to loss of melanin and cause pale patches of skin called vitiligo. If the fracture is worse and the immune system is in poor condition, not only do the stem cells flip the genetics of the melanocytes into cancer cells, but also the uptake of stem cells into the flow of the cerebral spinal fluid can transport these pseudo-antigens to the surface of the brain. Stem cells may attach to blood supplies in the brain and form brain tumors.

By itself, melanoma rarely causes death by destroying a patch of skin. Only when advanced melanoma metastasizes and spreads to vital organs such as the lungs, heart or brain does the melanoma pose mortal risks. Is it possible that arch and pedicle fractures can bleed stem cells into the spinal cord fluid, and on the ascending flow, find their way into sympathetic nerves? Humans can live a long time with a portion of skin not functioning properly, but we cannot go long without lungs and heart. Most death derives from respiratory failure. Dermatologists can determine with high certainty if a discolored section of skin is a harmless mole or a sign of melanoma. A technique known as epiluminescence microscopy uses oil on the surface of the skin combined with brightly lighted magnification to examine the skin. Even more accurate is a skin biopsy.

Fall Off Ladder Leads to Melanoma and Brain Tumors

Nancy, a patient of mind for over twenty years, told me of an interesting story while I treated her for lower back disc protrusion and leg pain. She reminded me of Jack, a retired tow truck driver who had moved to the state of Oregon. She told me he was ill with melanoma on his back, as well as brain tumors. Jack came into town several months later, and I was able to observe the melanoma cancer. The dark lesion was on his upper back to the left side over the spine.

An X-ray examination showed a mild lateral compression fracture on the same side and site of the lesion, and a possible arch fracture. I asked Jack if he had had an automobile accident or a fall before the melanoma had appeared. He reported that he had fallen from a ten-foot ladder and landed onto the ladder, striking the back of his neck and upper back. The fracture likely leaked stem cells that initiated melanoma in the skin; migrating stem cells flowing in the cerebrospinal fluid had found their way to the brain and formed tumors.

I have many living patients who have pigmentation patches that darken every year. Several of these patients had spine injuries earlier in life due to heavy work on a dairy. Some of these patients with pigmentation changes over the left side of the first two lumbar vertebrae ended up with colon cancer. The mutagenesis is different in time and evolution with each individual. A couple of individuals who fractured the lower right side of their thoracic vertebrae had rapid development of pancreatic cancer. Another individual who crashed his auto into a ditch off a freeway crushed all three of his upper lumbar vertebrae and was diagnosed with multiple myeloma within a week of his injuries.

Several patients I have been treating for pain and degenerative disc syndrome have mild pigmentation patches adjacent to one side of the spine that may signal the onset of melanoma or bowel cancer. These patches, two to three inches in diameter, show yellow or brown darkening to the side of the vertebrae. The vertebrae below the skin lesions have had a compression injury or a vertebral disc herniation. Because of the history of similar patients, I watch these skin color changes with great care. If the skin condition worsens quickly, I encourage patients to seek a biopsy and determine if they have melanoma or bowel cancer.

Remember the earlier story of Marilyn, who worked on the family dairy ranch for decades, and came to me for years of treatment after a life of working with cows and farm animals. While working with cows in a muddy pasture, she had slipped and fallen numerous times. Marilyn had a light brown pigmentation patch above the left side of the first two lumbar vertebrae. The pigmentation lesion became mildly darker as she approached the age of eighty. In her mid-eighties Marilyn was diagnosed with colon cancer.

It may be possible that other skin lesions begin with stem cell bleeding. Some 98 percent of people carry the herpes virus that causes shingles, lip blisters or other skin conditions. Herpes viruses, essentially packages of DNA, come in eight different versions that cause a variety of symptoms. Often the virus supposedly hides nearly undetected in the sacrum and cranial bone regions of the spine. If an accident causes a compression fracture to the sacrum or tailbone, herpes virus can leak out and result in an outbreak of shingles. In such cases, the virus may not have come from outside the body via exposure to another source. It may have come from the body's own stored virus, a dormant stem cell, before it was released.

I have seen numerous patients who developed shingles along a spinal level nerve or cranial nerve where there was a previous spinal injury. Several patients who had upper neck injuries developed facial shingles that coincided with the side of injury and subsequent vertebral subluxation. Patients with injuries to their thoracic vertebrae may also develop shingles at the level and side where their vertebrae were previously injured, and experience chronic vertebral subluxation. Shingles of the sciatic nerve down the back of the leg develop most commonly on the side of a disk lesion or chronic subluxation.

Most of the individuals I have observed whose traumatic spinal fractures evolved into cancer very quickly had poor immune systems, poor diets, and were not fed colostrum as an infant. Alcoholics and individuals who abuse prescription or illegal drugs have poor immune responses. A liver weakened by prolonged use of blood thinners cannot keep up with supplying the tens of thousands of proteins needed by an immune system that is fighting leaked stem cells. Skin cancers are highly associated with immune-suppressant medications. People who routinely take drugs to reduce the chance of organ transplant rejection commonly end up in a battle with skin cancer. Most relapses of skin problems, such as shingles, appear in patients who suffer from stress, poor diet, or repetitive spinal trauma.

SHINGLES AND DERMAL NERVES

In shingles, our immune system attacks the myelin coverings of dermal branches to the skin of our body and face. This immune response may have its start from trauma and resultant stem cell leakage. The immune response may be the producer of the viral proteins of herpes. In certain stages, herpes is contagious, but the virus may be derived from our own body due to an attack on the myelin that covers nerve pathways in the skin.

With the initiation of shingles as a process driven by stem cell leakage, secondary antibodies produced may be the culprits in the disease. Instead of stem cells entering the center of the nerve and migrating to the organ, the attack is on the covering of the nerve, and antibodies produced from this initial attack flow into the axon or center of the dermal nerve. Once antibodies reach the distal end of the nerve, shingle lesions erupt. Shingles, the usual manifestation of the herpes virus in dermal nerves, appears in the worst injured areas of the spine and the nearby exiting nerve. My patients who had a history of sciatica in the posterior of one leg had their outbreaks of shingles in that leg, but not in the other leg. Thoracic lesions also developed to the side of the ribs and spine where the vertebrae were previously injured. Facial shingles and Bell's palsy may erupt on the cranial nerve side where the upper cervical vertebrae have had past injury and subluxation.

In the fetal development of the spine, leftover embryonic stem cells are normally capped off inside the vertebral bodies of the spine. The segmental or somatic development of body organs and tissues are derived in memory chips called stem cells. Vertebrae at different levels house different stem cell codes from the ones above and below. Release the viral stem cells from one vertebral body through the center of the disc and into the one above or below and you get a myelogenous brew. Stem cells attaching to stem cells can produce multiple myeloma and leukemia. Multiple vertebral plate fractures typically occur before the cancer. Chapter 11 with discuss the outcome of multiple vertebral fractures. The relationships are there, I don't believe doctors are interested in the cause of illnesses. Doctors just don't ask the right questions and they don't investigate past possible spinal trauma.

CHAPTER 9

Multiple Sclerosis and Aortic Aneurysm

• • •

MULTIPLE SCLEROSIS IS A DISEASE where our immune system attacks and deteriorates the protective insulating covering, called myelin, of our nerves and spinal cord. Spinal cord images and tissue findings reveal scarring — sclerosis— of the coverings due to our immune system destroying myelin connective tissue and laying down scar deposits. Researchers recognize the autoimmune attack, but they do not know the exact cause or trigger for the disease.

Multiple sclerosis is generally believed to be an autoimmune disease. Our immune system that normally protects us against foreign bacteria and viruses, and cleans up protein waste products, is attracted to the myelin and begins to attack and dissolve it. This exposes the nerve — like an electric wire without a covering. The nerve's conductivity is compromised without its covering and it fails in its communication. Removing the covering of nerves produces symptoms of muscle imbalance, muscle system weakness, and feelings of aching and burning throughout the muscle system.

Neurological losses from multiple sclerosis can be intermittent or permanent. The disease is not as prevalent in countries located close to the equator, perhaps due to more sunshine and Vitamin D. However, these countries are less developed, with fewer transportation accidents, and do not have the ice and snow that lead to many injuries from falling that are common in countries in colder climates. Some studies look for a genetic predisposition to multiple sclerosis and try to identify a protein factor that is present or missing. It might prove beneficial to study whether or not an individual who develops multiple sclerosis had received colostrum at birth. Colostrum supplies many protein growth factors whose absence may make a person more susceptible to multiple sclerosis, as well as other maladies.

Other studies look for viruses as a link to multiple sclerosis but can't explain where they originated. Researchers are trying to identify antigens, or protein markers that attract white blood cells into action against the myelin covering. Interestingly, stem cells are not ordinary cells; according to research, they cannot be tagged due to a lack of surface proteins. Could it be that marrow stem cells penetrate the myelin when they escape a vertebral fracture? Could it be that the presence of stem cells attracts and trigger the immune system to attack the myelin coverings of the nearby nerves and spinal cord? Could these stem cells have leaked from a vertebral body fracture or a vertebral arch fracture?

AUTOMOBILE ACCIDENTS LEAD TO A LOW-GRADE MULTIPLE SCLEROSIS

Becky and Monica suffered similar types of accidents: they were stopped in their cars, and another automobile struck them from behind. The force of impact was moderate, but sufficient to snap their heads backward over

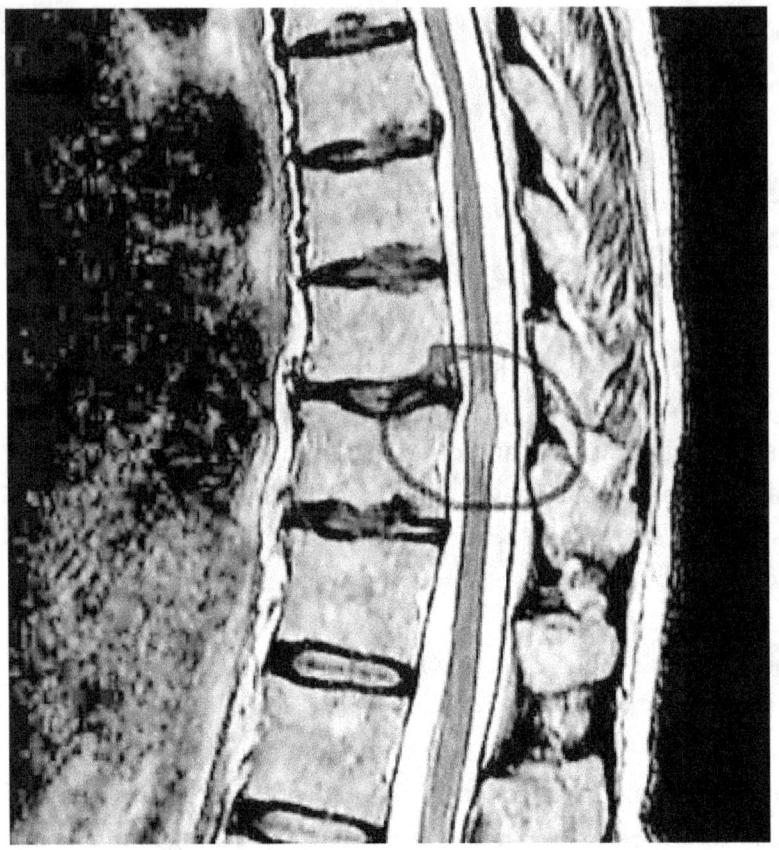

the top of the headrest. Their necks were over-extended backward and then immediately compressed to the lower neck vertebrae. Such compression to the back portion of the vertebrae can fracture the supporting arch and joint pillars.

Arch fractures are not commonly looked for by doctors and are typically detected only with skilled X-ray techniques that include lateral and oblique views. An arch fracture is located just behind the exiting spinal nerve root and close to the dorsal nerve root ganglion. Bleeding stem cells from this type of fracture could easily enter the myelin sheath of the nerve root or spinal cord.

Becky and Monica both developed burning pain in one shoulder and the scapular muscles on the same side. The pain, burning and muscle weakness appeared several weeks after the initial accident and lasted for over a year. In each case, an MRI of the neck was taken after two months of diffuse pain and weakness, which places the test at about ninety days after the accident. The MRI in both cases revealed sclerosis-type plaque or scar tissue inlaid at the lower portion of the cervical spinal cord on the side of the injury. Coordinating the MRI with oblique X-rays revealed pillar-type fractures at the lower cervical or upper thoracic vertebral levels. Stem cells may have bled into the nearby nerve coverings or spinal cord, and these stem cells may be the antigen or protein that attracted the immune system to attack the myelin, thereby triggering multiple sclerosis.

The initial arch fracture would have triggered an immune response, but why do some accident victims heal better than others? Many factors can disrupt healing ability. At the very beginning of the immune response, applying heat can swell nerve tissue to twice its size according to MRI studies. Could the application of heat force out even more stem cells from the bone marrow?

A person may face greater risk of developing multiple sclerosis and have weaker healing response if his or her immune system is compromised key factors: whether or not the person was colostrum-fed as an infant, and whether the diet is complete in sulfur-containing proteins. Does the person smoke? Is the person diabetic? Is the person a vegan or vegetarian? Is the person on medications that disrupt essential protein processing within the liver, which therefore thins the blood of available healing proteins?

A person with comprehensive healing ability can battle a transitory sclerosis condition to where the symptoms are decreased, and the disease is lessened. Others have poorly developed or over reactive immune systems that produce constant antibody proteins that signal the immune system into continuous action against connective tissues. Tissue destruction can go on indefinitely because the antibodies that are produced are genetically close to both the cells of connective tissue and the marrow stem cells that trigger their production.

Larger burst-type vertebral body fractures can bleed stem cells into cerebral spinal fluids. Stem cells need blood supply to evolve, and the spinal cord has a rich supply. Ironically, the immune cells produce the very antibodies that they in turn must conquer once the antibodies attack their own connective tissue cells. Inflammation breakdown products or proteins can be measured in cerebral spinal fluid for multiple sclerosis. Normally there is very little protein and few cells in the cerebral spinal fluid. An increase in certain proteins or immune cells can indicate autoimmune attack or other diseases. Abnormal protein levels in the cerebral spinal fluid can indicate damaged nerve tissues. Large levels of proteins in spinal fluid may indicate inflammation, tumors, or bleeding after trauma.

A compression fracture in the thoracic or upper lumbar region may allow the concentration or buildup of protein in the blocked or slowly ascending spinal fluid. A spinal tap immediately after a vertebral body fracture may indicate whether marrow stem cells have been released into spinal fluids. Reviewing hundreds of X-rays and MRI under the internet search of multiple sclerosis about 90% of the views revealed a single level vertebral compression fracture or posterior arch compression injury. The single vertebral body fractures were adjacent to the sclerotic changes in the front or anterior spinal cord. On side views of the neck region, the posterior arch compression type injury revealed sclerotic changes at the posterior portion of the spinal cord.

Neck compression injuries with hyperextension of the head, arch the neck backward and crush the arches of the vertebrae. Stem cells leaking from the posterior portion of the vertebra flow toward the exiting nerve roots and posterior spinal cord. This includes the dermatological branches that terminate in the base layers of our skin. Posterior bone marrow bleeding also allows cerebral spinal fluid to carry the genetic strips up to our brain. Depending on the strength of one's immune system, the stem cells will invoke the immune system to attack the brain coverings and cause myelin and connective tissue damage by auto-immune disease. Or with final failure of the immune system, the stem cells become cancer stem cells as they mutate the connective tissues of the brain into tumors and cancer. In any case, a very healthy immune system is crucial to conquering bleeding stem cells.

In the study of aorta aneurysm researchers found it to be an autoimmune syndrome. The same process of the immune cells attacking, disrupting, and devouring the connective tissue layers of the large artery leads to tissue disintegration and expansion. Hence, the artery dilates and expands. What I have witnessed in a dozen or so x-rays I have taken that contained an abdominal aorta aneurysm involved a lateral injury to the left side of the

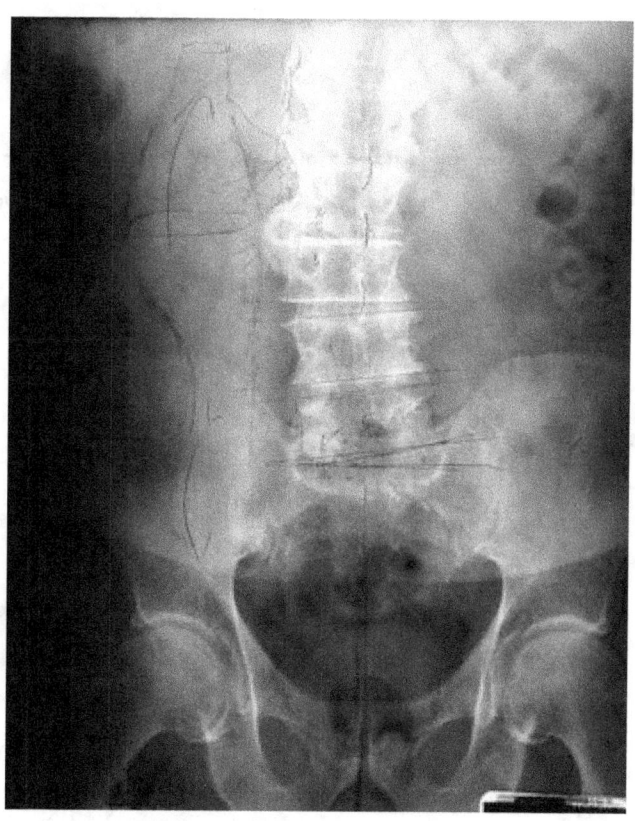

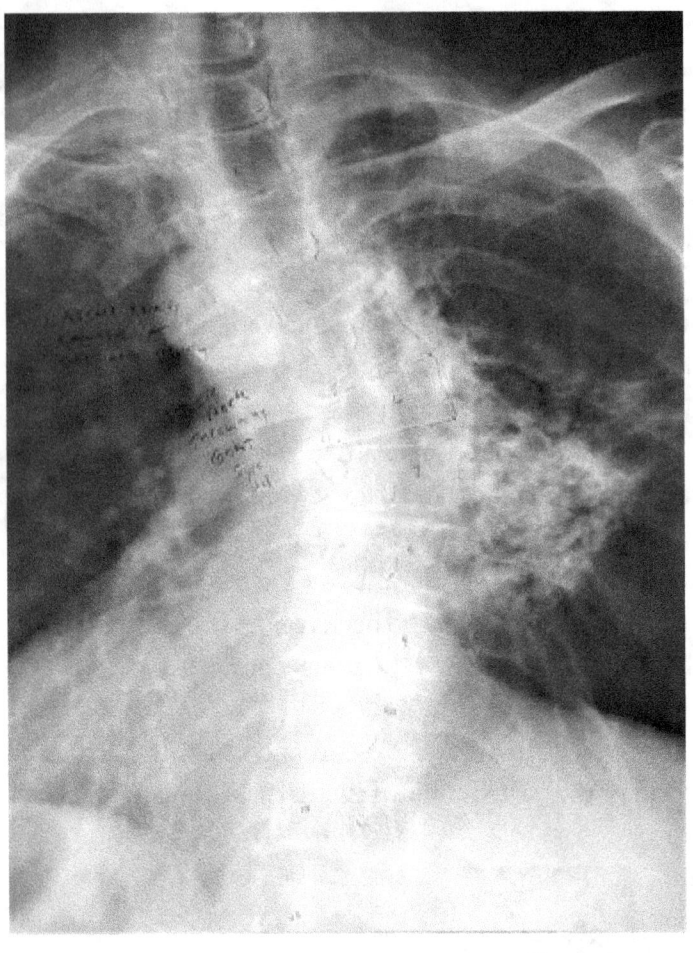

lumbar spine. The corresponding calcification or expansion of the aorta is always adjacent to the injury site. One day I read an article in a professional journal on aorta aneurysm and it contained an x-ray picture. Not surprising, the image of the lumbar spine had the same lateral injury at the site of the widening of the aneurysm. I believe stem cells bleed from the lateral type trauma and flow into and through nerves and ligament tissues adjacent to the descending aorta.

Injury at the thoracic spine on the left side will affect the thoracic aorta. Some of the trauma to the spine may have been fierce enough to affect the aorta itself. And the hundreds of x-ray images with small calcific changes seen in the medial wall of the aorta have an adjacent lateral disc herniation or vertebral plate trauma. A rib fracture near the spine can affect the tissues right beneath it. Like the earlier story of the woman who fell, landed on an object, and fractured a rib behind the heart. It led to a sarcoma change in her heart muscle.

Trauma to the spine produces changes that are local to the tissue region and to the sympathetic or parasympathetic nerve pathways from that level of the spine. The images I have viewed revealing MS, aorta aneurysm and ankylosing ligament calcification have always had a history of trauma. Most of the illnesses arrived weeks and months after the injury. The time factor in post injury illnesses are relative to the intensity of the injury and whether the person was colostrum fed. Every person's body reacts a little different to injury. The variables are due to diet, stress, immune system efficiency, medication side effects and other medical iatrogenicies. The spinal injuries seem to heal rapidly and efficiently during the time of puberty and growth hormone production. I find less cases of injury with cancer and autoimmune disease outcomes with teens going through pubescence and spinal growth periods.

CHAPTER 10

Medications, Osteoporosis, and Spontaneous Vertebral Compression Fractures

• • •

NON-TRAUMATIC VERTEBRAL COMPRESSION FRACTURES ARE not the main subject of this book; however, thousands of spinal fractures everyday are due to thinning and aging bone. The production of internal strands of collagen to build new bone may decrease with age, but millions of people are also thinning their bone as a side effect of medication. Emergency rooms everywhere see spinal compression fractures caused partially or entirely by blood thinning medication, and also by drugs aimed at building bone. According to news items about a year ago, Fosamax and Boniva may lead to fractures of bone. How could that happen? Your liver releases tens of thousands of tiny protein molecules into your bloodstream every millisecond. Good protein eating habits help your liver produce important building blocks to be sent out to your cells. Unfortunately, almost any medication you take has an ill affect on your liver's protein production.

JUST STANDING UP LEADS TO COMPRESSION FRACTURE

One Saturday afternoon I received a call at home from Fred, a 75-year-old patient I had treated for several years. Fred was anxious and in moderate pain, so I drove to his home with my portable table. I discovered he was in severe lower thoracic spinal pain and spasm. He informed me it started the hour before when he stood up from a seated position. I performed some light spinal muscle work, set him up with home ice therapy and worked above and below his segmental pain. I told him he may have had a spontaneous compression fracture of his thoracic vertebra. Fred had recently been prescribed blood thinners. I told him an X-ray would be important to look for a compression fracture of his spine. I instructed that he not lift anything and support himself when he gets up and down from a chair.

That Monday, Fred's pain had decreased from the treatment and using ice therapy. I positioned him for a standing

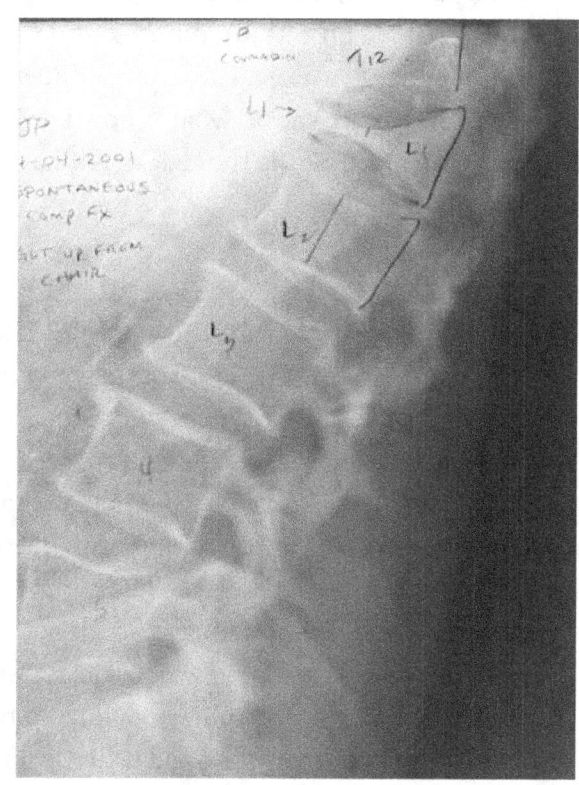

X-ray and noticed his posture was leaning forward. The X-ray revealed a moderate anterior compression fracture of his first lumbar vertebra. Fred came for treatments over the next four weeks. Unfortunately, a month after the compression fracture, he became very ill. Within two months of the injury, Fred passed on. His cause of death included respiratory failure. Nearly all his systems had shut down. The fracture location and the physiology of bleeding stem cells into Fred's organ systems may have triggered an overwhelming immune response that compromised his health.

Multiple Compression Fractures; First Six Months on Coumadin

Rose was a lifetime resident of our town and still worked in real estate sales into her early eighties. She was petite, vivacious, and always a pleasure to work with. One-week Rose called and was in serious mid-back pain. She had gotten up out of her chair at work the week before and felt mild mid-back pain. It progressively worsened so she called her medical doctor. X-rays revealed a mid-thoracic anterior compression fracture. By the time Rose called me, another compression fracture had occurred at the vertebra below the first fracture.

Rose was hunched over and could not straighten up. During her appointment, Rose confirmed she had been on Coumadin for only three months when the fractures began. As with other similar cases, the initial first six to 12 months on blood thinning medication often prompt spontaneous compression fractures. Patients on blood thinners for over one year have less chance of a bone-thinning fracture. Rose's health became very frail after the initial fracture, and she passed on within six months.

Considering that most elderly people succumb with respiratory failure, I have a hunch that some of that population had a thoracic compression fracture. A fall to the hip, slip in the tub or just getting up from a chair can lead to an unnoticed thoracic or lumbar compression fracture. I know of many elderly people, who after a fall, passed on within a month or two. Yes, they may have been in frail shape, and even a hip fracture is difficult for an 80-year-old. I still wonder how many seniors had a vertebral fracture that went undiagnosed. These fractures can lead to what is now known as a Catastrophic Immune Response where the red marrow leakage is too great for the thoracic or lumbar cavity to handle. The heart, lungs and organs are vastly affected and soon fail.

Picking Up Lawn Mower Compresses Lumbar Vertebra

Harold was an 85- year-old do-it-yourselfer who loved his home garden. He found his way to my office after he received unsatisfactory treatment from another chiropractor. Harold had severe pain in his lower back and along the sciatic nerve of one leg. A week before, he had bent forward to lift and move his lawn mower. He had been on blood thinning medication for about a year. I took standing X-rays of his lower back and before treatment. The X-rays revealed a fifth lumbar compression fracture that was underneath the vertebral body and more posterior --at the back of the vertebra. It also had part of the bone protruding backward like an open drawer. The protruding fractured piece was about half an inch out extending toward the spinal nerve roots.

Harold received treatment with spinal settings and long axis traction; he responded well. X-rays two months later revealed that the protruding bone piece had returned to position and healed into place. Harold received support chiropractic treatment and did well until a few years later. On one appointment he described getting up and feeling moderate upper back pain. He was X-rayed by his medical doctor; a thoracic vertebral compression fracture was found. Harold's respiratory system was never the same after the upper back fracture and he soon passed on.

Cancer patients on chemotherapy, steroid medication and radiation treatment develop iatrogenic bone thinning. Vertebral compression fractures that were present before treatment are subject to further bone weakening and deeper fracture. The new treatment of pumping a hardening gel into the center of the vertebral body— called kyphoplasty or vertebroplasty — may help pain and spinal posture but has its own side effects. It can lead to vertebral compression fractures of the vertebra above or below the procedure. Bone normally has malleability or flexibility, and any harder substance placed up against it can fracture the bone. I worked with several patients where the kyphoplasty procedure led to an adjacent compression fracture inside one month of the procedure.

Another procedure that failed with serious side effects years ago was the injection of papain enzyme into the center of a herniated disc. A problem occurred where the acidic enzyme would enter through the vertebral end plate and dissolve the internal bone marrow. Deaths that ensued were similar to the cases above where a portion of the marrow substance had been forced out through compression.

OSTEOPOROSIS AND VERTEBRAL COMPRESSION FRACTURE

Even though this book involves primarily trauma related vertebral compression fractures, osteoporosis is the predominant cause of these fractures. The disease starts within the structure of the trabecular cancellous bone in the vertebral body. The trouble lies in the inner bone matrix and lack of collagen protein strands being produced. There are reasons of age, activity, diet, disease, medications, and hormonal problems that can affect the inner bone matrix activity. I will not elaborate on the disease and hormonal aspects of bone loss. Most readers of this book may still believe that spinal cancer occurs before any metabolic bone loss, hence fractures are due to cancer. I do believe we live in a time where medications, processed foods, low essential sulfur protein uptake in the diet are some of the big culprits in osteoporosis populations. Decrease in bone density occurs in a percentage of men and women after age 40, and the process is greater in women who have undergone menopause. Populations of osteoporotic people who have a vertebral compression fracture are at

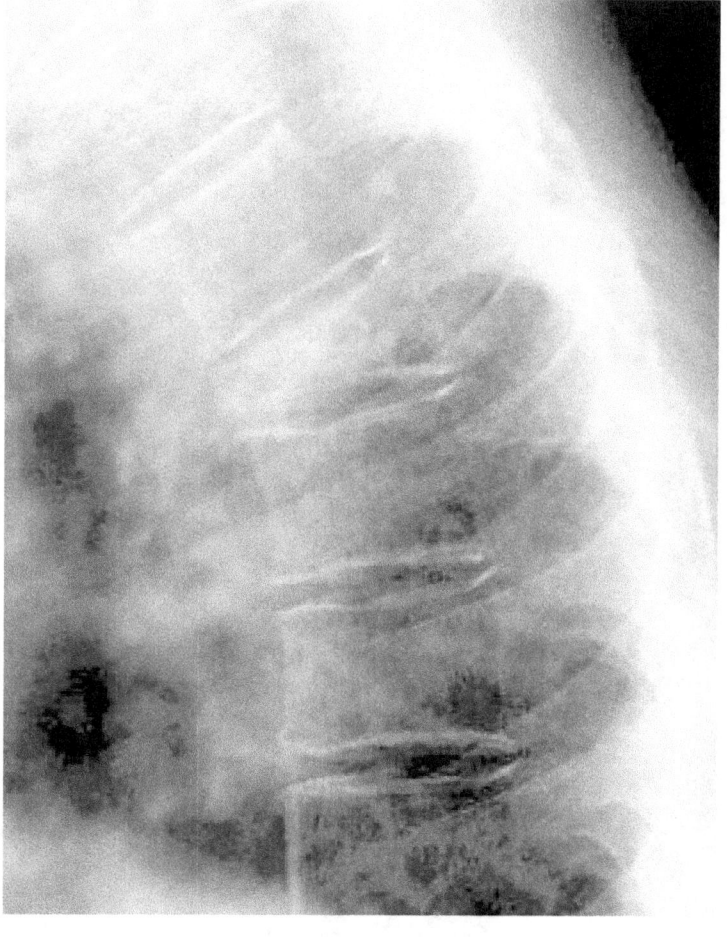

higher risk to have a second one. This group also has risks of leg and hip fractures. Above, I recommended doctors to always examine the spine for compression fracture when a fall and hip fracture has occurred.

Osteoporosis is a bone-weakening condition where the vertebral structures cannot withstand normal amounts of pressure or strain. As a result, the smallest of movements such as bending over, turning quickly, lifting even light objects, sneezing, and coughing can cause a vertebral compression fracture. Traumatic injury caused by a fall from a height or a motor vehicle crash can cause compression fractures, but a portion of the fractures can occur just standing up from a seated position. The lack of spinal muscle strength, restrictive spinal joint movement, and imbalance of muscle tone control can contribute to osteoporosis of the spine. Other risk factors that effect the inner bone matrix of the spine include tobacco use, alcohol consumption, vitamin D and calcium deficiency, inefficient uptake of essential sulfur protein, estrogen imbalance, and the lack of physical exercise, which is essential to activate the growth of the collagen proteins strands.

On studies of osteoporotic fractures, researchers never give a history of injury or medications taken. The Ph.D. scientists always recite the need for calcium, Vitamin D, and hormone balance when it comes to bone growth and strength. What is always missing is the fact that collagen protein strands are laid up and down and across the middle of bone before mineralization occurs. Sulfur proteins are essential in the diet for bone to grow and become flexible, as opposed to brittle. People who have a diet complete with the essential sulfur-containing amino acids make the proper connective tissue proteins for forming collagen and internal bone. Chapter 14 will discuss these essential amino acids in greater detail along with other enzymes that promote faster production of healing proteins.

CHAPTER 12

Multiple Myeloma and Leukemia

• • •

OUR CIRCULATING BLOOD SYSTEM CONTAINS plasma or blood cells that mature within our bone marrow from stem cells. Red blood cells, white blood cells and platelets develop inside our bones before they are released into the vascular system. The originator cell is known as a hematopoietic stem cell and is more like a small package of DNA than a cell. Through several histological stages, the stem cell develops into a mature blood cell. Disease occurs when marrow stem cells develop abnormal blood cells. What sets off this strange growth of cells is unknown, but it involves genetic change to the stem cells. Changes occur in the cellular DNA. Why mutations in a place where the cells are so protected? Myeloma and leukemia are diseases associated with such marrow alterations.

Multiple myeloma is a debilitating malignancy that is part of a spectrum of bone marrow diseases ranging from monoclonal proteins of unknown significance to plasma cell leukemia. Myeloma is a proliferation of irregularly developed and malfunctioning blood cells within the bone marrow. Cells multiply uncontrollably and are known also as cancerous plasma cells. First described in 1848, multiple myeloma was characterized by a proliferation of malignant plasma cells and subsequent overabundance of monoclonal proteins known as antibodies. An intriguing feature of multiple myeloma is that antibody-forming cells — the plasma cells — are malignant and produce unusual lineages of strange antibody proteins.

The proliferation of abnormal plasma cells in multiple myeloma interferes with normal production of blood cells, resulting in leucopenia, anemia, and thrombocytopenia. Cells gather in small soft tissue masses within the bone marrow, and these cells eat away the bone. Myeloma produces lytic or dissolving lesions in the vertebrae of the skeleton. Symptoms of multiple myeloma are bone pain, hypercalcemia, renal failure, and spinal cord compression. The aberrant antibodies that are produced lead to impaired immunity, and patients have a high incidence of infection, especially with encapsulated organisms such as pneumococcus. The overproduction of these antibodies may lead to hyper viscosity and renal failure. Systemic ailments include bleeding, infection, and kidney disease, and secondary pathologic vertebral body fractures.

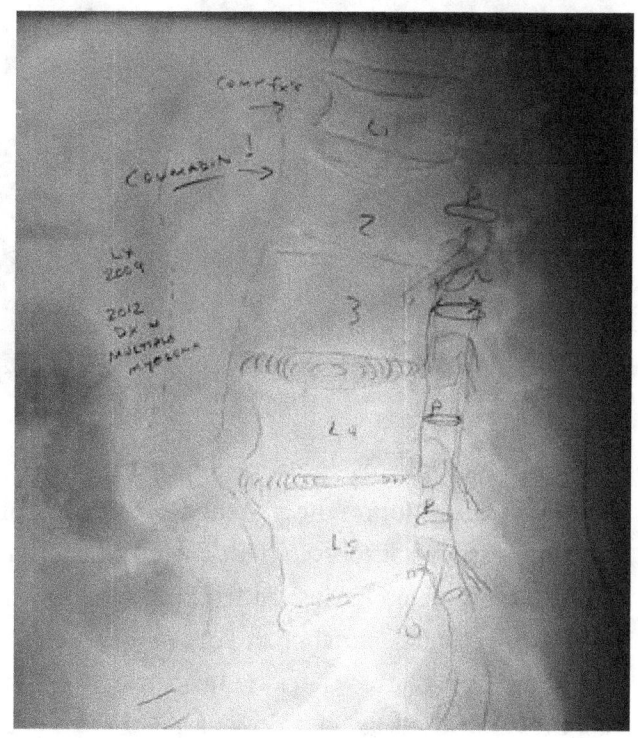

MULTIPLE VERTEBRAL COMPRESSION INJURIES LEAD TO MULTIPLE MYELOMA

The cause of multiple myeloma and leukemia is unknown, but the red marrow stem cells and their irregular divisions are known to be responsible. What is not known is how the blood stem cells suddenly become genetically irregular and flip over to cancer cell production. Is it possible that injury to the end plates of vertebrae allow stem cells of one vertebra to migrate into the marrow of another vertebra and set off a malignant marrow brew? Is it possible that the inherent stem cells of one vertebral body are somatically distinct and different from the stem cells in adjacent vertebrae? If so, are normal developing blood cells infected by the stem cells of a different neighboring marrow?

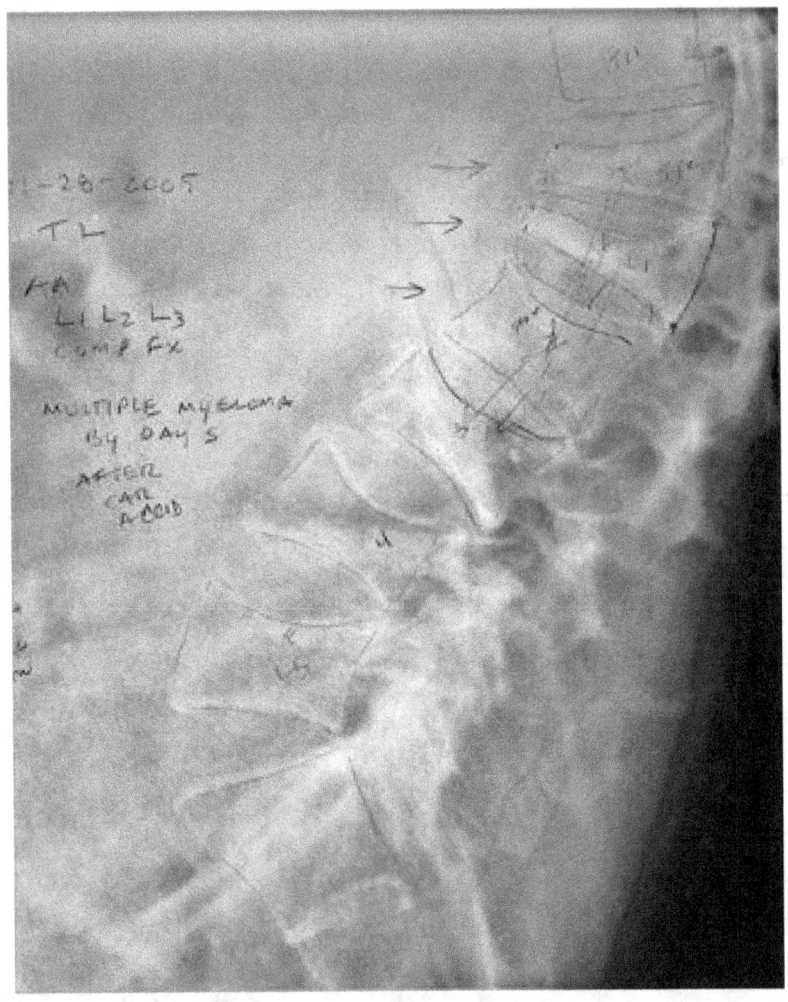

Tim was an experienced truck driver and delivery driver. Six years ago, in his early fifties, he was returning home from work in San Francisco when he lost control of his automobile in the rain. Tim's car spun and slid off the freeway, crashing into a culvert and hitting a cement wall. Because his older model car had no air bag protection, the impact of the accident pushed his body forward and down. It was a severe accident. Emergency room doctors took spinal X-rays and revealed multiple burst-type fractures of his first three lumbar vertebrae. Hours after the accident, Tim became very ill. Within the first couple days of the accident, Tim developed and was diagnosed with multiple myeloma. He had never been ill or diagnosed with multiple myeloma until immediately after the accident.

Roy was a top athlete in his youth and played several sports including football, basketball, and baseball. He had played through college and beyond. Roy was an avid golfer. When I heard he was suffering from multiple myeloma, I wanted to learn more. By the time Roy had reached his mid seventies, he had suffered from multiple myeloma for a couple of years. He allowed me to review his condition and study his X-rays and MRI images. I found the punched-in vertebral plates of his lower back very interesting. They appeared more like compression fractures and included both top and bottom end plates. In discussing possible related sports injuries, Roy revealed having landed on his tailbone many times, especially during basketball games.

Max was a cattle rancher and drove his truck through the hills and rough terrain outside our city every day. One late evening, after checking his cattle, the rain was coming down so strong, his visibility was challenged. Max drove off the road and down an embankment into a large crop of rock. The impact shoved his head and upper body toward the windshield. The fierce impact compressed his spine. Max ended up with vertebral compression fractures to two adjacent vertebrae. It occurred at the level of his first and second lumbar vertebrae, L1 and L2.

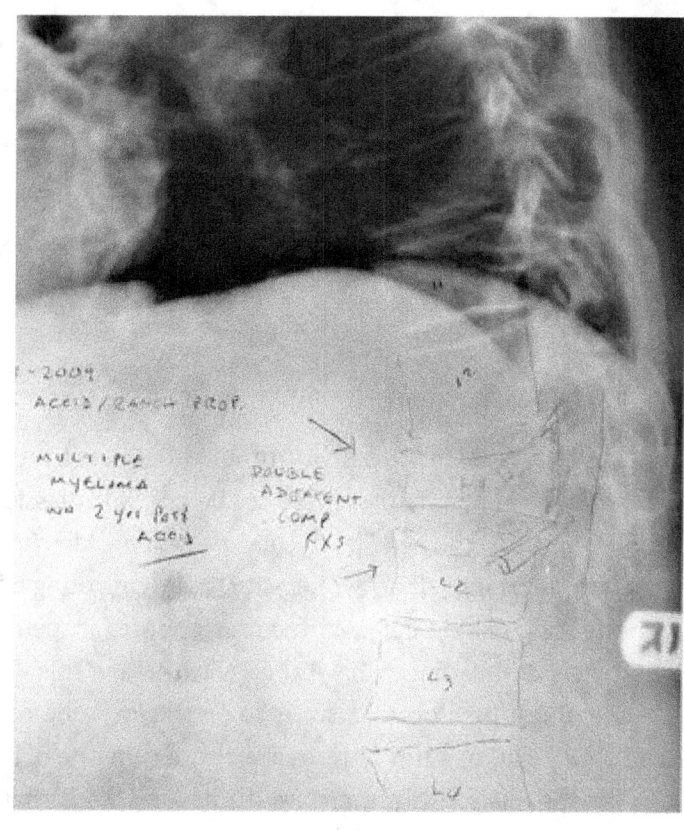

Max found his way to my office for lower and mid back pain and restriction weeks after the accident. I took x-rays of his spine to locate the levels of fracture. Treating him with spinal muscle massage, light spinal manipulation above and below the fractures and flexion traction was beneficial for his pain syndrome and healing. After a couple of weeks of treatments, I examined Max once a month for three months. About four months after I last examined him, I heard from other patients that he was diagnosed with Multiple Myeloma. This didn't totally surprise me, but it reinforced my idea that adjacent vertebral compression fractures lead to an intermixing of one somatic level of stem cells with stem cells from a different somatic level. The DNA blueprint of two differing stem cells produces leukemias and multiple myelomas. I realize most views on vertebral compression fractures are due to the evolving diseases, but in my experiences, this is not true.

I found a 2011 video clip of a radiologist from a spine treatment center discussing vertebral compression fractures with an athlete who competed in kayaks down vicious river rapids. Over several years, his patient received six vertebral compression fractures, at different times during his competition. The patient developed multiple myeloma after receiving these fractures. Did the compression fractures lead to the multiple myeloma, or did this incredibly strong athlete already have multiple myeloma and then the impacts of the kayak racing were too much for his weakened spine? I believe that trauma to multiple vertebral end plates allows intermixing of marrow stem cells from one vertebral body to another by passing through the center of the intervertebral disc. The stem cells are inherently different and may set off an intramedullary immune reaction that causes genetic changes in the blood cells. In bone marrow transplants, the treated individual has marrow cells of his own bone, or another donor, replaced back into his marrow system. Interesting, the person treated has all his marrow irradiated, hence removing the stem cell codes of all his somatic spinal levels. I only know one individual who received a bone marrow transplant. It may have added a few months to his life, but the suffering was worse. Bone marrow transplants are known to be very risky and do lead to the development of new cancer.

CHAPTER 13

Cranium and Brain Trauma

• • •

SOME SCIENTISTS STUDYING BRAIN TRAUMA have set a hidden agenda for the truth of their findings. This has been proven by the lawsuits presented on behalf of professional sports players. How fragile is the brain? Could one simple impact to the head lead to a variety of problems? Do multiple low-grade impacts to the upper body shake the brain tissue into disarray? Recent studies on young beginner football players has revealed brain changes even without concussion injury. With contact sports, it seems that each subsequent year of playing can further contribute to brain damage. I have already witnessed this with several athletes.

One question I found answers to on the internet, regards head trauma and location of a brain tumor. Can a head injury lead to a tumor formation under the site of impact? It can, and even though I found medical research refuting the relationship, there are studies and blogs that show it to be true. I dedicated the revision of this book in memory of Phillip. My life has come full circle, and my loving companion is his mother Isabel. I first met Isabel twenty-four years ago when she sought care at my chiropractic office. Over those initial years I told her of my ideas of spinal trauma and the possible relationship to cancer development. Then one visit she told me the sad news of her son Phillip and his health on edge with a brain tumor. Isabel knew of my ideas of trauma, and she told me of an early head injury Phillip had as a four-year-old child. Phillip had slipped head first onto the bottom of the bath tub and struck the right side of his forehead. As he rose up from the fall and impact, he was dizzy and fell again. He again struck the right side of his forehead. Isabel said he recovered fine, but several years later Phillip had a major seizure. On examination and imaging, doctors found a brain tumor under the location of his original impact to his forehead.

A brain tumor forming in ten-year-old Phillip was a life changing event for him and his family. Could stem cells at the location of the cranial impact have bled into the brain tissue and seeded a tumor? Isabel brought Phillip into my office when he was thirteen years old. I took x-rays of his head and neck and treated him for uncomplicated cervical subluxation. He passed away after brain tumor surgery at age fourteen. In my research concerning location impact and tumor formation, I found the personal blogs of brain tumor patients to be most interesting. They believed their injuries led to the development of their brain tumors, even if the doctors educated them differently.

There are several different ways tumors are seeded in our brains. Here is a sad story involving treatment of a child's brain with someone else's stem cells. You can find this story by an internet search by typing: Ten-year-old Israel boy brain tumors stem cells. You will find one of many stories of stem cell use in the brain that resulted in tumor type growth months after the injection. The progression of brain tumors in these cases were determined to be linked to the donor's stem cells. Donor's stem cells or our own red marrow stem cells can seed malignancies in brain tissue.

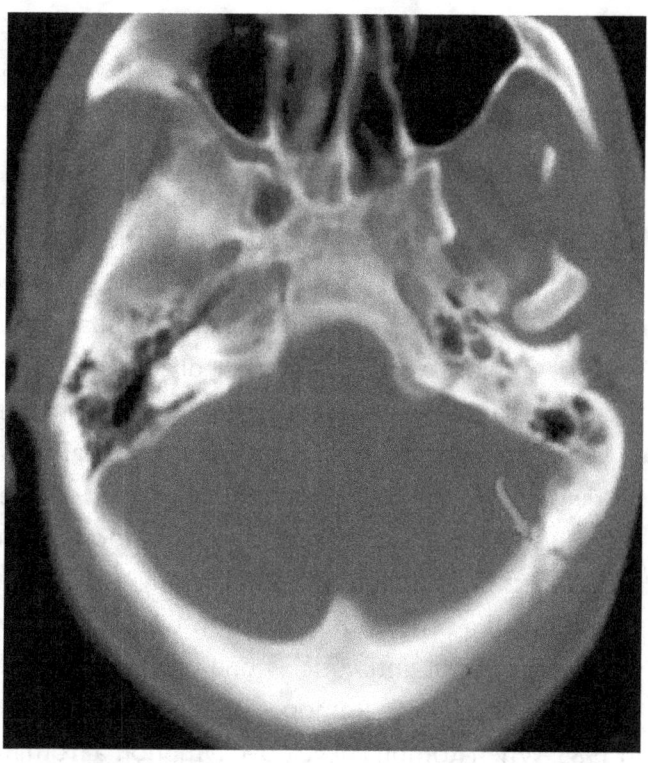

The cranial bones have an outer table of bone, a center intramural matrix of red bone marrow and an inner table of bone. On cranial impact, the inner table of bone can fracture inward, without fracture of the outer external table of bone. Unless imaged properly by x-ray, CT or MRI, the fracture of the internal table of bone will go undiagnosed. Internal cranial fractures can lead to bleeding onto the brain. A large bleeding can result in a hematoma or patch of blood and blood cells. The healing process of a hematoma with the infiltration of stem cells may develop different types of brain tumors depending on the site of infiltration into the brain tissue.

Cranial bone trauma and bleeding may be a cause for seeding of brain tumors. Another way stem cells enter the brain is via the circulation of cerebrospinal fluid. A crushing fracture to the vertebral body or posterior arch or pedicle can bleed out red marrow stem cells. The genetic material can penetrate the thecal sac and enter and follow the ascending flow of the cerebrospinal fluid. This clear, colorless fluid surrounds the brain internally and externally to cushion and protect the Central Nervous System. It bathes the brain and spine in nutrients and eliminates waste products. Most seeding of brain tumors occurs at the surface brain tissue, and not deep within. The presence of an immune response in cerebrospinal fluid may indicate an infection, but it may also be due to stem cell infiltration after a recent fall or spinal injury.

Brain trauma also occurs without stem cell bleeding. The fragile gelatinous brain tissue is 80% collagen tissue. The brain is disrupted and damaged by internal crushing due to sudden abrupt head movements. In a broadside automobile accident, an impact to the driver side door will relay a quick lateral force to the driver's head, abruptly moving the brain tissue within the cranium. Studies have proven that broadside impacts lead to a tearing deep down between the two hemispheres of the brain. Cognitive changes develop post head trauma. I have treated many automobile accident patients who could not return to work for months or years after brain trauma. I personally did poorly in my first two years in college, which followed the five-car pileup in my senior year at high school.

One moderate concussion of the brain can change a person's life forever. Other times, the head movements of smaller but repetitive impacts lead to brain dysfunction. Several patients I have examined regularly over a twenty-year period had brain changes due to their continual participation in contact type sports. Starting young in football, rugby, boxing, kick boxing, soccer and basketball can have an accumulated effect on the brain. Any sport that can lead to a head injury is a potential producer of later life dementia, cognitive problems, personality change, depression, and suicide.

In football, the terrible truth is revealing the curse of impact sports every week in the news. Football players of all ages and levels have developed brain problems. In later years, players who had several concussions have brains that are showing debilitating diseases including Dementia, Alzheimer's, Parkinson's, Chronic Traumatic Encephalopathy, Multiple Sclerosis, and Amyotrophic Lateral Sclerosis (ALS) or Lou Gehrig's Disease. Personally, I know of dozens of individuals from sports and head injuries who developed ALS. The cases I have seen, had probably head injury with the impacts to the back of the head. I believe red marrow stem cells infiltrate the cerebellum tissue by two channels. Many of the observed patients had a previous blow to the back of the head or occiput bone. It occurred due to sports or a backward fall. The other cases involved a fracture elsewhere in the spine or cranium, with the entrance of stem cells into the cerebrospinal fluid. Transplantation of stem cells into the cerebellar tissue produces an immune response against those tissues.

Our brain has an extra protective epithelial layer of cells covering the brain vessels called the Blood Brain Barrier or BBB. The BBB is thought to protect our neurons from bacteria and virus infections. Could it be that the BBB also protects the brain from infiltration of stem cells after a cranial trauma or bleeding? My wife Romona succumbed from lymphoma and brain lymphoma. It was like the way ALS patients deteriorated in the brain. Romona had a serious drug reaction to ciprofloxacin in 1989, which damaged her liver and nervous systems. Cipro, a powerful antibiotic, is one of the only medications that can pass through the blood brain barrier. I donated my kidney to Romona as a second transplant in 2002. She first received a kidney from her sister Monica in 1985. When Romona developed lymphoma from her immune suppression-antirejection meds, the lymphoma was able to pass through the BBB and deteriorated her brain.

I have seen the histories of individuals who when hiking had fallen backward striking the back of their head on rock; football players who have been struck in the back of helmet; auto repairmen, building contractors, and plumbers all who have struck the back of their heads on equipment; etc., etc. Many of these individuals developed ALS months or years later. Hyperextension neck injuries with lateral impact can collapse or fracture the vertebral arches or pedicles and can lead to MS, ALS, and brain tumors. Arch fractures go unnoticed all the time. The pain is the same and right next to facetal joint pain. Why is it that several of my patients and friends who crushed their necks developed brain tumors or esophageal cancer years later? Head injuries lead to eyesight problems, cranial nerve problems, and bipolar brain conditions. In any ten miles per hour automobile collision, a concussion is produced. The brain is certainly fragile!

CHAPTER 14

Colostrum: First Immune Codes

• • •

During late pregnancy, a concentrated fluid of immune proteins and their codes, gathers at the breast, ready for the baby's birth. Colostrum is known as first milk. It is thick and yellow, and available to the newborn for the first three to seven days. The all-natural substances in colostrum include immune factors, growth factors and tissue repair factors. Colostrum delivers nutrients in a very concentrated low-volume form. The newborn's digestive system is immature and porous. Colostrum helps act as a mild laxative to help the passing of the baby's first stool, which is called meconium.

Immune proteins, called antibodies or immunoglobulins, are present in this first milk. 70% of a human's immune system is gained by immediate ingestion of colostrum. They are quickly and easily absorbed, and travel through the blood to areas where they are needed for tissue protection and cell activation. Two of these areas are the lining of the airway to the lungs, and the lining of the digestive tract. These surfaces are important areas to be protected from immediate bacteria or viruses. The surface cells of the lung, where oxygen is exchanged, are not only protected by immune proteins, but are also prompted to function by proteins that allow the surface of lung tissue to open for the exchange of oxygen through lung membranes. These proteins are known as surfactants. A newborn's lungs are immature, and colostrum gives the child a better breathing start.

Antibodies contained in colostrum are produced based on the mother's previous experience with infections. Even the infant's grandmother's immune code is most likely passed on to the mother if she received breastfeeding. Immune protein codes that a baby receives are handed down from generation to generation unless a female baby does not receive the mother's first breast milk. These precious immune proteins are ready in the colostrum to provide passive immunity for the newborn. Humans are one of the only mammals who have a partial immune system working at birth. All other mammals do not have an immune system when first born and must receive colostrum to survive. Cattle ranchers and other animal farms defrost bottles of colostrum hours before a calf or animal is born. The application of colostrum must be done within an hour of birth. Having the colostrum ready saves the calf if the mother cow succumbs after giving birth.

Humans can survive without receiving colostrum, however, the non-colostrum fed population is lacking 70% of a proper immune system. In the 1950s, doctors and health care providers were told that breast feeding a newborn was not necessary. I believe this was a drastic end to long lineage of defense codes handed down from generation to generation. A lot of new illnesses appeared in the 1950s and now everyone had to get vaccinations to survive. How well does a vaccination work if you do not have 70% of your immune system to begin with?

One important question I have asked of most of my 5000 patients was–did you receive colostrum at birth? Interesting to find that those who did not, had an 80% finding that they were allergic to milk. Watching over the non-fed group, I found they suffered many more allergies and illnesses. In my studies on who developed autoimmune disease and who developed cancer after a marrow bleeding injury-the non-colostrum fed population were more likely to develop cancer post-injury. The colostrum fed population had an immune system that battled better, and illnesses initially remained as an inflammatory condition or autoimmune syndrome.

Immune components of colostrum include:

Lactoferrin
A protein that acts as an antioxidant, binds up iron from red blood cells that need recycling and helps prevent infant jaundice. Bacteria need iron to survive and multiply. Iron is not readily available when lactoferrin is present, as this protein binds, transports, and releases iron only to the body's own cells. Lactoferrin combines with other proteins to provide an antibacterial defense for the digestive tract.

Proline-rich Polypeptides (PRP)
These small immune proteins are sensitive to disease agents such as bacteria. They signal immune cells to turn up the attack on pathogens, and then signal the cells to damper or back off the attack. PRP reduces the frequency of oxidative or oxygen damage to the DNA of cells. PRP is also effective on disease states characterized by an overactive immune system, such as allergies, asthma, and autoimmune diseases. PRP has been studied in its effect to help neurodegenerative diseases such as dementia, and Alzheimer's disease.

Lactoperoxidase
An abundant enzyme in milk found almost exclusively in the whey after cheese making. Lactoperoxidase is a single chain sugar protein molecule made up of iron and calcium. It is an antibacterial agent natural to milk, saliva, and tears. The sulfur oxidation action by lactoperoxidase can chemically destroy bacteria and other microorganisms.

Interleukins
Interleukins are signaling proteins from T-cells that respond to increases or decreases of bacterial or cellular replication. Most interleukins direct other cells to divide and differentiate. They are like a dimmer switch on a light bulb, reacting when necessary to advance or withdraw an immune response.

Tumor Necrosis Factor (TNF)
Macrophage and monocyte immune cells produce TNF, a multitasking protein that directs and signals other cells to start growing in large numbers or self-destruct. TNF can cause tumor reduction by cell destruction and bleeding. TNF is a major director of cytokine production during inflammation. Overproduction of TNF is associated with the development of several diseases, such as rheumatoid arthritis, Crohn's disease, atherosclerosis, psoriasis, sepsis, and diabetes.

Cytokines/Chemokines
Cytokines are messenger proteins produced by cells. They communicate with cells of the immune system to regulate responses to disease and inflammation. Some cytokines stimulate production of blood cells. Others

help cells grow further and enhance their abilities. Some are involved directly with the immune system only and attach to white blood cells to direct the immune response.

Chemokines are like cytokines except they work further away from the lymphatic system to carry a signal to recruit leukocyte immune cells into action.

Growth factors in colostrum include:

- Gut-transforming factor
- Insulin growth factor
- Platelet growth factor
- Fibroblast growth factor
- Epidermal growth factor
- Vascular growth factor

All these factors and more are involved in giving the baby codes for proteins to initiate and continue proper protein production for protecting the digestive system, promoting blood sugar uptake in cells and muscle, formation of healing and mending proteins such as platelets and fibroblasts, and lifetime generation of cells that need constant replication, such as the internal digestive lining, skin, hair, and blood vessels.

The connection between infant breastfeeding and a child's subsequent health is well-known. Here are some infant risks associated with not breastfeeding a baby:

- Infectious morbidity
- Otitis media/ear infection
- Respiratory tract infection
- Gastrointestinal infections
- Obesity and metabolic disease
- Neurocognitive development/I.Q.
- Sudden infant death syndrome/SIDS
- Infant mortality
- Dermatitis
- Asthma
- Type-1 Diabetes
- Childhood cancer

All these risks of not breastfeeding have been researched, and there are likely still more health risks to be discovered. Studies on the outcomes of mothers who had breastfed a child have shown reduced chance of breast and ovarian cancer, and diminished risk of obesity later in life.

Colostrum has amazing lifelong benefits when provided at birth. What about the population of people who never received this first vaccination? If a mother skips a generation of breastfeeding her daughter, would the daughter's colostrum be as adequate from her generation on? Is it beneficial to consume colostrum as a protein food or immune support aid as an adult? More research must be done. Since the 1980s, I have been asking my patients whether they were fed colostrum. If stem cells migrate untouched through sympathetic nerves and end up in the support tissue of an organ, would a person who had received colostrum have a better chance at controlling and eliminating the foreign stem cells? I believe so.

I have observed distinct differences in those who did or did not receive colostrum at birth. Those who did receive first milk have a healthy immune response that can conquer the entire situation of leaking stem cells, or the stem cells are conquered enough by a sufficient immune system to allow only an autoimmune disease at the site of the stem cell entrance. Patients of mine who were not colostrum fed and suffered a lateral vertebral fracture had a higher incidence of cancer with early diagnosis. Some patients who developed cancer months to years later prove that our immune system can win or lose the battle at any time. It is amazing how our bodies can go through so much and still function for another day. There are a few studies which conclude that colostrum may help prevent osteoporosis in adults. Since breastfed babies have more growth and healing factors since birth, as adults they have a more robust system to ward off the most destructive intruder of all — their own stem cells. Stem cell research has found that certain individuals have a protein that slows or prevents cancer stem cells from activating the gene that promotes their profligate dividing. Could it be that those individuals received the protein through colostrum feeding? More research needs to be done on the differences of healing ability between those who have or have not received colostrum at the onset of life.

CHAPTER 15

Prevention and Immunotherapy

• • •

ESSENTIAL SULFUR AMINO ACIDS

THERE IS A BOND, a common thread that makes up all living things. In fact, it started eons ago with bacteria, and is found in all living cells. The miracle of life began with the bonding of carbon to sulfur. Even though the double strand of DNA structure has four repeating protein codes that do not contain sulfur, the sulfur to carbon bond and crosslinking has given rise to billions of genetic codes since life began. Life of even the smallest bacteria are all due to the bioavailability of bonding sulfur and other minerals to carbon. It may have begun with rainstorms washing out inorganic sulfur into the oceans. Sulfur in water allowed the first formation of living cells. Without organic sulfur, there would be no life on earth. The connective tissues of our body are made of collagen proteins.

Sulfur-carbon bonds are flexible and elastic. Hence collagen is also elastic protein: keratin, or elastin. Collagen fibers and cells are the aging tissues of our body. They are constantly growing and replacing themselves. The connective tissue collagen forms the framework of all organs, bones, vessels, and skin. Collagen protein is the flexible glue that holds all forms of living organisms together. Mineralized collagen makes harder tissue, such as bone and teeth. Connective tissue includes ligaments, cartilage, hair and nails. Some collagen is highly organized, such as the eye, which allows light to pass through. Some collagen is less organized, and allows movement and flexibility, such as ligaments and tendons. The collagen proteins of all living things are the same. We have a common thread with all living things.

Proteins are threads of molecules. Minerals combine to make the structure of molecules. Minerals are bonded to carbon atoms to make living structure. Sulfur-to-carbon bonding allows molecule motion or elasticity. DNA and all living matter are here because of sulfur-carbon bonding. The double-helix protein strand of DNA and its dividing properties are due to sulfur. Collagen protein is made from sulfur amino acids, the building blocks of proteins. The generic name for collagen is "glucosamine sulfate." Organic or dietary sulfur is needed to support protein and DNA replication. Our connective tissue system is a collagen-based system and includes the immune system. The strongest and most virile animals eat only the organs and connective tissues of their prey. There is a huge collagen protein deficit in the American diet.

Our body has amazing form and structure that is adaptable and resilient. We have a connective tissue system that is elastic and endures a wide range of motion and injury. The specialized cells of the body rely on cells that can reproduce rapidly and maintain form. The common thread in all connective tissue is a sulfur-based protein called collagen. They can be called glucosamine sulfates, but let's tag them as sulfur proteins or collagen. The miracle in these structural proteins starts at their molecular level where carbon bonds to sulfur. One researcher has noted in an article about this bond, every living form on this earth relies on sulfur and its bond with carbon."

The bond is elastic and allows architectural freedom. All form and structure of tissues and organs are set in place by collagen fibers. Skin, the largest organ, is about 75 percent collagen. Our heart contains 30 percent collagen, the liver 40 percent. Brain cells are held in place by a collagen matrix that makes up 80 percent of the brain. Organs such as the colon and intestines are composed of 25 percent to 30 percent collagen.

Bone begins as 100 percent collagen until it is mineralized with calcium. New internal bone growth is undergoing a constant change. Collagen strands of protein are laid down for new bone as other cells remove bone. Your bone today is not the same structure that it was a year ago. This is the same for your hair and nails, which are made of keratin protein, a sulfur protein.

The connective tissue system is also responsible for the form and production of blood cells. Red blood cells, white blood cells and platelets are built from sulfur proteins. Organ systems produce proteins in the form of cells, hormones or organelles that move through the vascular system. These proteins are primarily structured with sulfur. Soft tissues and organs are formed with 20 percent to 30 percent collagen. Ligaments and joint cartilage are formed with 80 percent to 90 percent collagen when water is removed. Sulfur-related protein is the most abundant protein in the body. Collagen fibers are in production constantly. Red blood cells are produced at the rate of two to three million cells per second. Sulfur proteins in our joints or vertebral discs reproduce at a very slow rate. Collagen cells placed in a petri dish with nutrients, along with vibration motion, produce 10 times more new fiber cells than cells that are not moving. Sulfur proteins make up the slimy slippery substance of mucous which lines the digestive tract and the nasal and airway tracts. Saliva contains immune cells which are made from base proteins of sulfur.

Because sulfur has a vital relationship with protein in our body, sulfur-containing amino acids, the building blocks of proteins, are essential to health. Several amino acids are categorized as "essential amino acids" in that they are not reproduced in our own body. This means they are raw materials needed for the body to survive. The DNA structure that forms a double strand of protein and divides into two relies on the bonding ability of sulfur. Without the building blocks of sulfur amino acids, we would not be here.

The vital four amino acids that are sulfur-laden are methionine, taurine, cystine and cysteine. These amino acids are needed on an hourly basis to allow the body to function properly. Foods containing these essential building blocks will be listed later in this chapter. Sulfur is the most important mineral in the body other than carbon, which is the foundation mineral. Sulfur is involved in the formation of B vitamins, thiamin, Vitamin C, biotin, hormones for metabolism, and coverings of healthy nerves. Sulfur plays a role in allowing cell walls to be permeable for the process of breathing, exchanging oxygen and cellular products.

Sulfur proteins are involved in energy production and carbohydrate metabolism. Sulfur is a significant component of insulin, the protein hormone secreted by the pancreas that pulls sugars into cells. Lack of sulfur amino acids in the diet can result in low insulin production, which can lead to diabetes. A diet high in sulfur protein and low in sugar might increase the body's ability to produce insulin to the point where insulin injections can be reduced.

Absorption of nutrients in the intestines relies on a healthy bile system. Bile contains the sulfur-made immune cells that pick-up nutrients. Mucous production in the stomach to protect it from digestive acids is dependent on sulfur amino acids. Immune cell production of proteins called antibodies in reaction to injury and infection relies on adequate intake of sulfur proteins. Coverings of our nerves and brain are called myelin sheaths, also made of sulfur proteins. Substances made by nerve cells called neurotransmitters need essential proteins to allow the nervous system to perform properly.

People want beautiful hair, skin, and nails. But more important, most would prefer a life free of pain, and longevity that is healthy and disease-free. The breakdown of collagen becomes a protein of pain. Smashed, broken-down sulfur proteins are known as inflammatory proteins. They are absorbed into tiny -fibers that signal pain. Inflammation products also absorb into nerves and tissues and are the cause of neuritis and immune system reactions that cause illness and suffering. To have a proper healing system, one needs an adequate intake of sulfur amino acids daily.

Organic or dietary sulfur is a mineral and does not cause an allergy reaction. It is considered nutritional. Sulfur is needed for many enzymatic reactions and is involved in all protein synthesis within cells. It is necessary for the formation of numerous different collagens of the connective tissue system. It is present as keratin in hair, skin, and nails. Sulfur from cysteine and methionine amino acids work with insulin to regulate carbohydrate metabolism, aid liver processes by helping glutathione production and work with glucose-amino glycans to help with joint cartilage and the linings of joint capsules.

Sulfur is also important for cellular respiration. It is needed in oxidation-reduction reactions, allows permeability of membranes that help cells use oxygen and uptake water, and in release of waste products. Several studies have shown effective uses of sulfur for problems of chronic inflammation, allergies, hyperacidity, and chronic constipation. Sulfur extracted from the sap of trees in the form of methylsulfonylmethane (MSM) can be used internally or externally for sulfur-deficiency diseases and degenerative collagen diseases such as osteoarthritis and rheumatoid arthritis. MSM is considered safe and non-toxic. There is no specific RDA for sulfur or sulfur-bearing amino acids.

To absorb nutrients in the body we need sulfur amino acids. Foods high in sulfur include: eggs, poultry, milk, milk products such as cottage cheese and whey, organ meats, gelatin, cartilage, fish, shellfish, broccoli, cabbage, Brussel sprouts, asparagus, kale, turnips, garlic, onions, and cooked dry beans. Seaweed, kelp, and blue-green algae also contain sulfur. Do you eat the skin of chicken? Do you savor another animal fat that contains collagen? Do you chew the cartilage off the end of bones? Do you cut up bones and boil them for soups?

There are plenty of dietary sources of sulfur proteins. Each person can find an ample source. Sulfur is available as a dietary supplement in tablets and capsules. However, you most likely do not need to take extra sulfur. If you are eating a well-balanced diet that includes adequate sulfur protein, you should be getting all the sulfur you need to maintain your body's daily functions. When a lion, tiger, wolf, or other predatory animal makes a kill of another beast, it first consumes the viscera: organs, lungs, heart, and tracheal tubes of its kill. Viscera are composed of collagen proteins, laden with sulfur amino acids. Even a grizzly bear consumes the skin, organs and eggs of the salmon and throws the meat and bones aside if salmon are plentiful. Consuming the connective tissues of other animals is better for us than just consuming the muscle, or meat.

The muscle or meat of animals is composed of a protein structure that is more nitrogen based. Meat, the center portion of muscle minus the tendons, is only five percent collagen. Is any meat from animals a good source of sulfur protein? No. Beef may get some bad press, yet chicken muscle fibers are no different. Is eating only meat a source of quality proteins? No. It is not a sufficient source of sulfur proteins. Plenty of other amino acids in meat may be important, but not as important as essential amino acids containing sulfur.

Muscle cells do not replicate or make new fibers. You are born with a permanent set of muscle fibers. Muscle cells need nutrients and energy, but they do not divide into new cells. Muscle fibers are formed of nitrogen-based amino acids that contract. Meat consumption in excess leads to an increase of waste products of nitrogen such as blood urea nitrogen. Urea is formed when meat proteins are broken down during normal metabolism. Excess urea is converted into uric acid, overworking the kidneys. Uric acid accumulation in the far extremities leads to gout. Joints at the ends of the extremities are lacking in sulfur proteins and overburdened by waste products of meat proteins. This leads to painful degeneration of the joints in an area where it is difficult to maintain circulation.

Where meat consumption may lead to systemic problems, consuming collagen-based proteins will not. However, the first question I get after presenting information at lectures on things to eat for sulfur protein regards cholesterol. Since lipoproteins, especially high-density types, are derived from sulfur proteins, you consume the good with the bad. Most people who have become allergic to shellfish and other foods were able to eat them for years until they digested them while taking an antibiotic. A poor overworked immune system can't process protein when carbohydrates and medications are consumed.

Inorganic or non-dietary sulfur in medications, antibiotics and preservatives can be detrimental to your health at a dosage only your body knows. Sulfa drugs, sulfates, sulfites, and sulfides are found in medications and foods that disrupt the smallest level of protein production. DNA and its repeating codes of organic sulfur proteins are not able to utilize inorganic sulfur, and the immune system reacts to this. Allergic reactions can occur to these types of inorganic sulfur compounds. While your digestive system absorbs a sulfa drug, the absorption of other proteins you have previously been sensitized to can suddenly cause an attack by your immune cells. If your immune cells produce a response with an antibody to this normal dietary protein, you have now become allergic to a food you never had a problem with before.

Sulfides and sulfites in wine and all kinds of preserved foods can cause the same allergic response. They are close, but just distant enough from our own sulfur-based DNA that the immune system overreacts at times. Another example of closeness of DNA is consuming one's own collagen proteins. This problem was identified in bovine spongiform encephalopathy, known as mad cow disease, and noted in a study involving chickens. If an animal consumes a large amount of its own connective tissue protein, it can form an antibody against the protein. This antibody then attaches and disrupts normal collagens of its body, and the immune system attacks normal connective tissue of the brain and nerves. This leads to failure of the nervous system and death. Consuming organs or tissues of your own species can be hazardous to your health!

Organic or dietary sulfur is approximately 0.25 percent of our body weight. A 160-pound man has less than a half pound of sulfur as body weight. Sulfur originates in the ocean and reaches the human food chain through rainfall. Sulfur protein availability is lost from food by processing, drying, cooking, and preserving. Sulfur proteins play a major role in operating and promoting numerous body functions. They are responsible for the elastic bond between cells and tissues. In tissue healing, immune cells produce type 1 and type 2 collagen fibers to provide cross-link repair of injured tissue. Cells are dividing 24 hours a day, and proteins by the thousands are released into circulation every millisecond. Studies on sulfur deficiency reveal slow wound healing, scar tissue overdevelopment, brittle hair or nails, gastrointestinal problems, arthritis, acne, and depression.

Our body is in a constant state of breakdown and repair. It needs raw materials to maintain healthy cells. Without sulfur amino acids the body will produce weak, dysfunctional cells. Cell death releases irregular and waste proteins that plague our body systems as free radicals. Sulfur proteins are non-allergenic and non-inflammatory and have no interfering or undesirable effects on medications. You cannot overdose with dietary sulfur, as the body will use what it needs and flush the rest without harm. These proteins also function as scavengers of free radicals and foreign proteins, and they clean the bloodstream so allergies to foods or pollens can be reduced or eliminated.

There are many ways to get adequate sulfur protein into your diet. One of the best ways to absorb sulfur amino acids and other amino acids is by consuming whey, a milk protein. Whey and casein proteins are the two primary proteins of animal milk. Casein protein comprises up to 70 percent of cow's milk and is used to make cheese. Casein protein does not contain the full spectrum of amino acids found in whey protein. Whey protein is extracted during the cheese making process. It can be dried as a powder protein and refined into concentrated amino acids. Human milk is approximately 70 percent whey, and 30 percent casein. Whey protein is nearly complete in total amino acids and amino acids containing sulfur, where casein is not. Cow's milk is 30 percent whey and 70 percent casein proteins, the inverse of the proportions in human milk.

The process of concentrating whey protein can denature or lose some of the amino acids and other immune proteins present in milk. I have interviewed hundreds of patients and people who have a milk allergy or intolerance. Of those who knew, 80 percent said they were not breastfed. More investigation needs to be done with people who did not receive protein codes provided by colostrum. The population of non-breastfed people has more difficulties in fighting and preventing disease.

Another important ingredient in collagen formation is enzymes or catalysts that assist in production of specific collagens. Each type of collagen in our tissues and organs is genetically different. There is similarity of course, however there are protein sequences at the ends of each type of collagen that make them unique. In nature, antioxidants are protein enzymes that help the collagen structure remain normal. Vitamin C, ascorbic acid, helps preserve healthy collagen proteins. So, does the antioxidant glutathione. But other antioxidants such as lutein and vitamin A help eye collagen and skin collagen, respectively.

Quercetin bioflavonoid changed my life 20 years ago when I added the supplement to my diet along with sulfur proteins. It was the only antioxidant I was taking. After two weeks my 25-year suffering from lower back and leg pain from a lumbar disc syndrome healed by nearly 98 percent. Fruits and vegetables contain all the antioxidants we need; however, manufacturers of vitamin supplements produce some natural and high-potency nutrients that will help you promote protein production.

To heal is to seal, and prevention of stem cell leakage or its consequences involves a healthy diet of essential proteins and antioxidants to fortify an immune system so that it is ready to respond. A first step to having a proper immune system is to promote first milk and colostrum feeding for infants. A study needs to be done on non-colostrum-fed people to find out what disease-fighting immune codes they did not obtain. Is there a different response to healing a vertebral compression fracture when the codes of colostrum were not present?

There are myriad ways to traumatize the spine. Preventing accidents through education and awareness should be a first step in reducing vertebral compression fractures. Safety in sportsmanship, wearing proper protective gear and informing youth of the risks of their sports will help prevent injuries. Wearing seat belts, knowing how to fall, and knowing which medications cause side effects of thinning bones will all help prevent spinal fracture.

IMMUNOTHERAPY

Besides the above, our biggest help will come from medical researchers and their production of reprogrammed stem cells and immune supportive proteins. Stem cells need to be genetically modified, so the immune system will not attack them. If the benefit outweighs the risk, stem cells that are genetically modified may be accepted in our tissues to make changes that will destroy cancer stem cells without damaging normal cells. Immunotherapy uses a person's own immune system to fight diseases, such as cancer. The proteins are engineered as antibodies to aid in activating our own immune system into operating better in attacking cancer cells. Research-made proteins can genetically alter one's immune system and deactivate cancer stem cells. While some therapies boost the immune system in a general way, others play out more specifically to attack cancer cells. Immunotherapy can be used alone, or in conjunction with other therapies. Attacking a specific part of a cancer cell can be done with monoclonal antibodies. These are lab produced immune system proteins.

My hope is that my theory presented in this book will prompt researchers to find more answers to questions on autoimmune disease and cancer. The family, friends, and patients I have cared for deserve to know how stem cells get into normal tissues and cells. Can a mild vertebral compression fracture lead to organ failure? After a compression fracture, can we safely test the spinal fluid for stem cell bleeding? Could we safely inject the red marrow of an acutely fractured vertebra with an irradiated tagged protein and follow it out into nerves and tissues? Can we safely medicate organs and tissues via the nerves, and to include the passage of modified proteins and stem cells to heal the tissues at the nerve-tissue junctions?

There are many ways cancer can start in the body. The American and Canadian Cancer Society's websites down play trauma as a cause of cancer. Scientists need to step away from their microscopes and scanners and get to know the individual patient's health and trauma history. Since I wrote Stem Cells and Spinal Trauma in 2013, I have many more stories to share. Patients with spinal compression injuries have come in this year who have been diagnosed with ulcerative colitis, systemic lupus, prostate cancer, acute pancreatitis, and colon cancer. I am still searching for people with fractures of the spine who have suffered subsequent illness. I shared the latest research articles on Facebook regarding the improper use of stem cell therapy. People offered information on their own compression fractures and illnesses such as lupus and endometriosis.

Recently I questioned local doctors and nurses about the possibility of a universal health record system for all individuals. I thought such a health record system was well into place. I found this situation to be put aside. I believe a computer programed system that kept an entire lifetime of an individual's health status, from the standpoint of vaccinations, medications, surgeries, injuries, and their outcomes would be a benefit to researchers. Or would it be? Seems this system was introduced years ago, but it has never really developed. Could it be that some of the outcomes of surgical or medication deemed to be failures would blemish the medical establishment? Maybe a comprehensive record of medical treatment outcomes would be too revealing and too forthcoming with the truth.

In 1985, I first theorized that stem cells were the culprits in autoimmune disease and cancer. My family, friends and patients have believed in my theory for almost three decades. I hope the stories in this book help you understand your illness, and you keep the faith alive and work with your medical doctor. I also recommend that you seek treatment with a chiropractor. A Doctor of Chiropractic can relieve pressure from an injured spine and allow it to heal more properly. Treatment can be focused above and below the vertebra that was fractured. Your chiropractor can help you with nutrition to help heal your fracture.

If you or a loved one fell ill after a vertebral compression fracture, please let me know. I may continue to revise this book with more pictures of X-rays and stories of bleeding spines. Many of my patients are living better lives thanks to medical treatment and natural remedies. There are incredible stories of cancer survivors and autoimmune disease victims enjoying a better life thanks to medical research. As I write, thousands of antibody proteins are being produced and tested by research science labs to tag cancer stem cells and attract our immune system into rendering them harmless. The greatest hope is that doctors and patients will openly share their own stories then ask new questions. How do stem cells of the bone marrow get painted into the picture of illness? Help us find the answer. If you suffer from any of the diseases or maladies described in this book, may you find renewed health, and may you live a long life free from pain.

Since a young child, I have had a passion for understanding the underlying cause of illness. I believed there was more to disease than microorganisms. Medical science has answered many questions on health issues the past hundred years. Many questions are still unanswered. Hope comes from understanding. Understanding illness and cancer takes time. Doctors and researchers will make progress. Maybe the ideas in this book will help. Thank You!

www.ingramcontent.com/pod-product-compliance
Lightning Source LLC
Chambersburg PA
CBHW081205180526
45170CB00006B/2226